I0118635

EASY QIGONG

a Silk Reeling Tai Chi warm-up routine

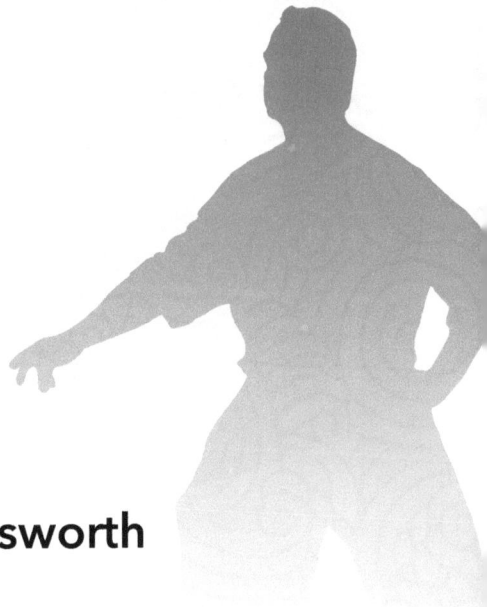

By Paul G. Ellsworth

Copyright © 2025 Paul G. Ellsworth

All rights reserved. No part of this book may be reproduced
or used in any manner without the prior written permission of the copyright owner,
except for the use of brief quotations in a book review.

To request permission, contact the author at Paul@PaulEllsworth.com

Library of Congress Cataloging-in-Publication Data: Ellsworth, Paul G.

Easy Qigong: a Silk Reeling Tai Chi warm-up routine / by Paul G. Ellsworth

1. Health and Fitness – United States – Handbooks, manuals. 2. Exercise – United
States – Handbooks, manuals. 3. Personal Health and Fitness. 4. Qigong. 5. Silk Reeling
Qigong. 6. Tai Chi Chuan 7. Tai Chi. 8. Martial Arts. 9. Flexibility. 10. Meditation. 11.
Stress Reduction I. Ellsworth, Paul G. II. Title.

ISBN 978-0-9710003-4-6 (6x9 version)

"Magic Light" by: Amaurie Ramirez
Website: Amaurierazphoto.com
Instagram: @amaurieraz
Movement photographs by: Marie Cetin
Website: MarieCetin.com
Instagram: @MarieCetinPhotography

Dedication

To Heaven, Thank you for the gift.

To Mom & Dad, for always being there for me.

To Sifu, for accepting me as a student & making internal arts real to me.

To those who wish to refine themselves.

To Taoists everywhere past & present

Acknowledgment

No book is written entirely in isolation.

Every author is supported and aided by others.

Thank you to my family, sifu (teacher), kung fu brothers & sisters,

my students, martial arts colleagues, & friends. However, without the

help of Gerald P. Ellsworth (retired USAF Major), and

Joyce C. Morris this book would not exist.

TABLE OF CONTENTS

PREFACE

The writing of this book of exercises initially began as a list created by my father. Over a period of some time, descriptions and explanations developed based on our conversations and training or practice sessions. This was intended to help my Dad remember this routine by having reference material when he was practicing on his own.

The primary reason for this was that we did not live in the same city. He traveled on business extensively. Our getting together for review on a regularly scheduled basis was minimal. I have felt and continue to do so that martial arts forms are the perfect traveling exercises available. The specific exercises laid forth in this book can be practiced anywhere where you can put two feet by anyone with a desire to do them. They can be modified to adjust to the needs of the individual.

> ## The primary purpose of this book is to facilitate the conditioning of oneself through whole body movement.

The formal name of these exercises as I was told is "chan ssi ching" or "tsan tzi chin" translated from the Chinese language into English as meaning "silk reeling spiraling power exercises." Apologies if I am spelling these words incorrectly from the original language. These movements are based upon the concept of the Circle and the ways the circle and curves appear in nature. These exercises are intended to help train and maintain the body, mind, and spirit to unify in all things done. It is my highest recommendation for the reader to seek direct training from a properly trained and qualified teacher. This text is intended to be supplemental to live teaching or direct learning experience. I have created a video series that is intended to be a companion to this book and for this book to be a companion to the practice and training videos.

I have been asked over many years by students and friends, "Could you or Would you write it down for us?" or "It would be nice if you wrote a book with these exercises in it!" Well, here it is! In my training we were not allowed to write or take notes while training or in classes. Additionally, video recording was not allowed either.

It is with my deepest, sincere respect to those teachers and experts who are familiar with "chan ssi ching" that I ask them to forgive me for what might be a simplification to their actual practice. It is not my intention to go into all the deeper internal energy attributes of these exercises in this book. It is not the purpose of this writing to go into extensive dissertation on the meditative, philosophical, spiritual, or martial application qualities of these exercises. It is my opinion that silk reeling qigong may be essential or enhance attaining higher levels or skill abilities of tai chi chuan for those seeking improved internal development regardless of style.

This series of exercises is my own interpretation of silk reeling qigong taught by many teachers throughout the generations, specifically as taught to me by my Sifu: Master F.J. Paolillo. His endorsement is not implied.

I recommend the reader review the written material prior to practicing any of the exercises. Reviewing the stances is specifically recommended as they are used throughout the routine presented in this book. What is done on one side of the body should also be done on the other side of the body. Do the same amount of exercise on each side of your body. If you do 8 counts or 8 rotations of circles with your left shoulder, then 8 counts or 8 rotations of circles should be done with your right shoulder. If you are physically unable to do the exercise in a low stance, it is recommended to only go as far as is comfortable for you until accustomed to the exercise. If you feel pain while doing these exercises, you are doing them incorrectly. This is not a "no pain, no gain" exercise program.

Additionally, independent practice of the stances will improve one's strength and quality of the other exercises. They can also be used as meditation postures. Familiarity with stances can only improve one's ability. These exercises were designed to loosen and limber the joints yet strengthen them such that the internal energy known as chi will circulate freely.

To keep this book to the point, I have omitted the discussion of chi development, which according to some qigong teachers will naturally develop through regular practice. Silk reeling qigong can be done without having to learn tai chi forms as qigong development exercises for those who choose to do so. They can stand on their own as they are excellent health exercises.

Paul Ellsworth,
Atlantic Beach, Florida
ending Year of the Wood Dragon, January 2025

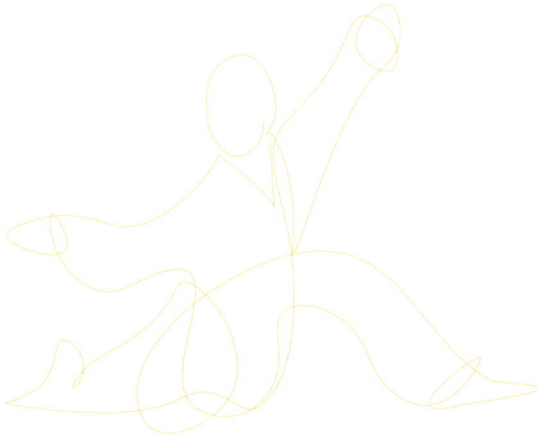

WHERE TO BEGIN
What is Qigong exactly?

Whether you believe in internal energy (chi) or not, this is what qigong (pronounced chee-gung) is supposed to encompass. Qigong is a holistic system that focuses on your posture, movement, and breathing, as well as key meditation practices. The goal is to improve your health, performance (specifically regarding martial arts), and/or enhance your spirituality. With origins that date back thousands of years, there is so much to learn and discover in terms of the history of qigong, how and why it is practiced.

The more you understand about this holistic system, the greater control you will have over each practice and the associated benefits. As you begin to better understand what this system is and how it is used, you can then implement what you have learned into your daily life and routine, hopefully benefiting you for years to come.

INTRODUCTION

Hi, I am Paul Ellsworth.

I have been practicing the Chen family style of tai chi chuan since 1991. These silk reeling qigong exercises were taught to me by my Sifu: Master F.J. Paolillo. He trained and learned them from Master Zhang Xue Xin. I use these silk reeling qigong exercises as a warm-up to my tai chi and kung fu practice. Those that have trained with me know that I just call them my warm-ups.

My opinion:

> **There is a wealth of knowledge behind what may appear to be a bunch of simple exercises.**

These techniques were developed centuries ago with the intention of improving internal vital energy and maintaining excellent health. I make no claims as to the validity of what they can and cannot do, except I feel better when I do them.

When doing the exercises the practitioner's focus and intention should be to facilitate the conditioning of oneself through utilizing their whole body in the movement.

These exercises or movements are based on the concept of the circle. The idea of the circle and the natural circular range of motion of one's body, and at the appropriate ability for the individual doing each specific exercise or movement. In doing these exercises some consider it to be a method to retrain and remind the body, mind, and spirit connection by unifying and linking or connecting in all things and ways of moving our bodies.

A benefit or value is these exercises require little space and can be done anywhere. It is my understanding they have been designed to limber the body and strengthen the joints as much as naturally possible.

According to some that believe in chi and the body's energy these exercises may promote the circulation of the internal energy known as chi.

Aside from being employed as warm-ups, these exercises can stand on their own. They can be used as conditioning exercises for anyone wishing to incorporate them into a regular exercise program. It is my opinion these exercises may be essential for higher levels of tai chi chuan training for anyone seeking improved internal development, regardless of the practitioner's style.

One of the main things when we are doing these exercises is that we want to be certain that the tongue is touching the roof of the mouth. This is like saying the letter L, such that the tongue should go up behind the teeth, but not touch the teeth. There is a slight gummy part in this region of the mouth, but the tongue stays up as long as you are comfortable doing this, and the breathing should be within or through the nose. The breathing should be from the lower abdomen area from within what some call the dan tien. The breathing should ideally be done so that you are inhaling up or in and exhaling down or out through the nose.

The mouth is kept closed during these exercises. The dan tian, for those that are not aware of it, is to be located about 2 or 3 fingers width below the belly button and inside the body. For me or from a western hemisphere point of view this would be our physiological center of gravity for our bipedal physical form body. Some claim there is a field of energy within this body area, some identify it as "the lower dan tien." I just simply refer to it as the dan tian.

Focus the mind's intention on this point within the body, the lower dan tian. I am suggesting that you want all your physical movement to begin from within this area of the body. When you begin by turning from your waist this way it will be seen visually. With time the movement should be less visible. However, to acquire that skill level may take years to accomplish the internal turning with imperceptible external observation. Part of the reason this is considered an internal martial art or training style.

One of the other things to remember as far as with the tongue to the roof of the mouth, is that from a very basic, practical point of view that tai chi chuan embraces martial arts in that if the tongue is sticking out and you get hit, you may end up biting your own tongue in the process of it so you don't want to stick the tongue out.

That is one of the very basic practical reasons that with the tongue touching the roof of the mouth, it keeps it in a safe place so that the teeth can be up. And of course, you do not lock your jaw or your teeth. The mouth and jaws should be gently closed. One of the reasons for having the tongue up to the roof of the mouth is from an internal energy point of view, this is connecting two of the prime meridians.

Now, I am not an expert in acupuncture or that type of topic. But, when the tongue is up from the way I view things, it is like electricity in a home. When the light switch is in the down or off position, technically there is electrical energy circulating in the house. And, when the tongue is up, this is like turning the electric light switch in a room to an "up" position. It is in an "on" position for connecting and linking active energy channels. This is connecting the electrical circuits within the body or the meridians.

It is activating it so that the energy or chi can come up from the earth or ground, and flow through the front of the legs. Going up through the dan tian and coming along and around the back of the body, continuing to come up through the top or crown of the head continuing down, dropping through the upper palate of the mouth. From there coming down the upper part or front of the body.

The tongue is the connector point. From that point comes down the front torso of the body and then it goes down the lower, back side of the legs grounding into the earth. So, energy can come up through the earth, through the body, around and back down.

The main thing is the dan tien is the collection area, the reservoir, the field of chi, the ocean of chi, where everything is gathered. And then from there, it all comes out. You have energy coming in from the crown of the head as well. The heavenly energy or the yang energy coming down, as well as the earthly energy or yin energy coming up through the feet.

Additionally, there is a concept that our body's skin can absorb air and water as a filter. There is a concept that breathing is from the inside or skin drawing energy into the body and expelling or pushing out on exhales. So, all points of the body, any surface area, can be breathing energy through the body.

For those that want more of a deeper energy explanation, the main thing that you want to do is when you are doing the exercises you want your feet to be firmly grounded once you are in place, sort of gripping to the ground.

FUNDAMENTALS

When standing upright with good postural alignment, be mindful to keep the knees slightly bent. The knees are slightly bent so that you can stretch the spine, so it is aligned properly without overstretching and not slouching. By doing this it allows for a spiraling or corkscrewing motion going down into the earth or ground, and a spiraling or corkscrewing motion going up to the sky or heaven. Be certain to maintain a relaxed, yet good alignment in the spine. The buttocks or the tailbone should be slightly tucked. Maintain awareness that the knees should be slightly bent so that none of the joints are ever locked.

There is always what I call natural extension or just a light bend at the elbows. You never lock the joints. It is a key rule. Never lock the joints. Ideally, the knees never go past the ball of the foot. They never go past the toes. And once you are in a position, make sure that what I call the rear foot or the rear heel of the foot stays down, be certain that the heel does not come up and down as you are doing motion such as when going forward and back the ball of the foot, and the knee does not go past the ball or the center part of the toes, and then the rear foot should stay firmly planted or rooted to the ground floor when you are going forward. So, you are rooting from the rear foot to go in a forward linear direction. The tailbone should be slightly tucked with the spine lifting the jawline.

Ideally, eyes should be level or horizontal, chin should be level, eyes looking forward horizontal. Then, if you need to check alignment, you could just look down. But wait. Now I realize something. Now the problem here is that my spine is out of alignment. So, you know, it is okay to look once or twice just to make sure everything is okay with the alignments when we are doing a sinking exercise. Eventually, you should be able to feel the alignment of the spine, crown of head, chin, chest, shoulders, knees, and feet without having to visually double check.

Ideally, if a person sinks down, almost sitting in an imaginary chair and can go to where the thighs are parallel to the ground, they could do that. This is excellent if able to do. But for many individuals, just sinking down a little is completely fine. You want to keep the tailbone tucked and the spine aligned, and the crown of head ideally would be upright; like an imaginary string gently lifting it up vertically. Ideally here the knees do not go past the toes, so you want to just sink or gently sit into the posture aligned.

Anything more than that is an unusual and unnecessary strain on the knees. The legs are just slightly below the full extension of range. So, there is always a natural bend at the knees. Be aware to never overextend.

AMBIDEXTROUS

Each of us as humans has a preference that does not always make sense as to where it developed or why we seem to unknowingly choose or lean into its usage regarding the use of our body. Examples of choosing between eyes, ears, hands, and feet.

Some individuals tend to have a more predominant right brain or left brain, and predominant right eye or left eye, and predominant right hand or left hand, and predominant right foot or left foot. Doing these exercises I believe will continue to develop the coordination of both sides of the body creating a better ambidextrous ability. I cannot prove or disprove this opinion. However, in my life experience I have developed some strong semi-ambidextrous skills or abilities. I give these exercises some credit. It is possible what I am describing was a natural inborn innate genetic ability and these exercises have helped to develop or maintain what I am suggesting.

> For consistency of doing these exercises and memorization of each sequence and to easily flow into the next exercise I deliberately chose to start each side with my left side and then complete with my right side and to remember to do both sides and to do both rotational directions of outside & inside, or clockwise and counterclockwise as appropriate for the specific exercise and part of the body being utilized.

> For consistency of the routine and its form memorization I prefer to start with an outside circle then change rotation direction to inside circle, then change sides and begin with an outside circle change the rotation of the circle to an inside circle. Continue by changing position to the other side to begin the next exercise.

note: for the left side of the body the outside circle will be in a counterclockwise rotation circle and for the inside circle it will be in a clockwise rotation circle. and in contrast: for the right side of the body the outside circle will be in a clockwise rotation circle and for the inside circle it will be in a counterclockwise rotation circle

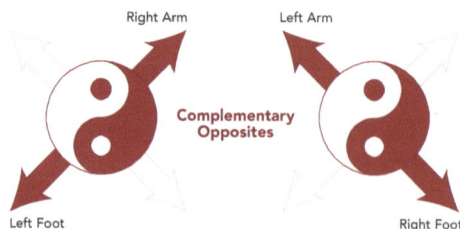

Right Arm   Left Arm

Complementary
Opposites

Left Foot   Right Foot

A QUICK PREVIEW

This is the general format or positioning of the body for each exercise except for standing in a neutral position

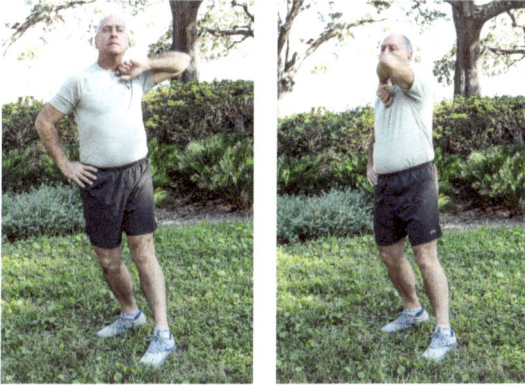

----- left side forward

Left Side
Outside Circle Rotation = Counterclockwise
Reverse the rotational circle direction
Inside Circle Rotation = Clockwise

Change Sides

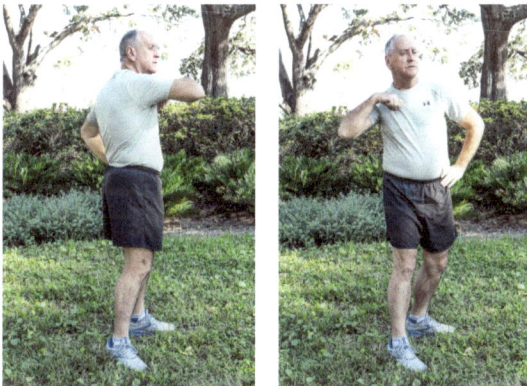

----- right side forward

Right Side
Outside Circle Rotation = Clockwise
Reverse the rotational circle direction
Inside Circle Rotation = Counterclockwise

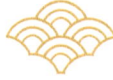

Before doing any of these exercises:

1   I ask that you read and re-read the names and the order of the routine a few times

2   Becoming familiar with what is going to happen in the sequence will help to remember them better

3   It all begins with starting from the head progressing through all the joints moving eventually to the feet

4   Please read the routine names and sequence order at least 2 times

Thank you

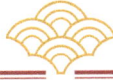

QIGONG ROUTINE

open with cleansing

picking fruit

head turning -
left & right, and head circle

shoulders

elbows

wrists - single & doubles

shake or stir the chi

cleansing

ward off & roll back

bend forward & pull back -
open & close

horizontal circle
single & doubles

hips

knees - individually

knees - left side
outside & inside circles
forward & back

knees - right side
outside & inside circles
forward & back

knees - together & knees apart

pick up ball

lifting while holding
the ball & circles

side tilt

pat shoulder

elbow to toe

polish the mirror

grind corn

look over shoulder

snake arm
single & doubles

shake or stir the chi

cleansing

3 standing meditation postures:
earth
sky-heaven
human-embrace

wu ji or wu chi meditation

close with cleansing

STANCES

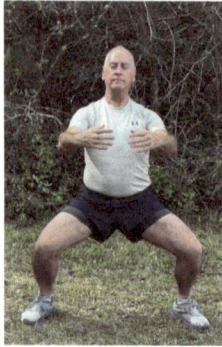
horse stance - embrace

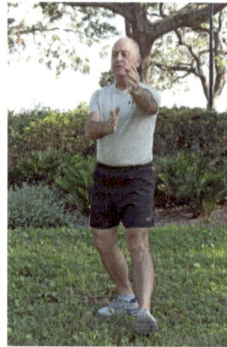
7 star - play guitar

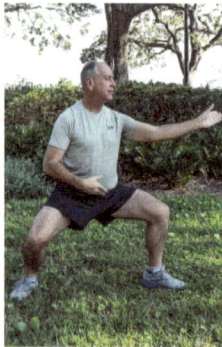
bow stance

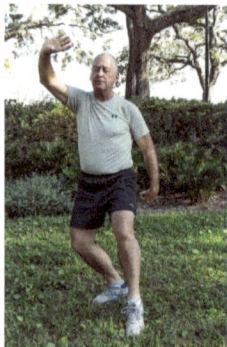
cat stance

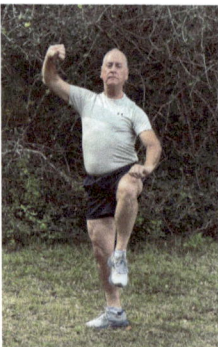
single leg

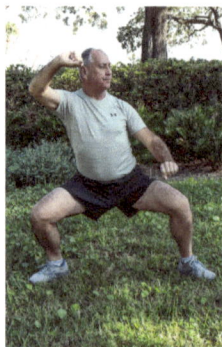
back stance

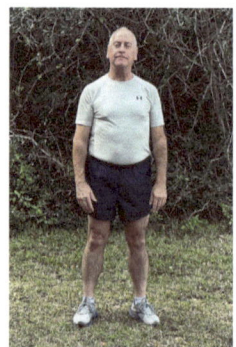
neutral stance

please read the above routine names and sequence order again at least 2 times

QIGONG ROUTINE

Here are photos in sequential order of the
qigong routine to help in visualization of doing them.

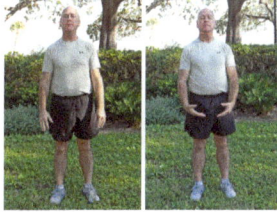

wu ji

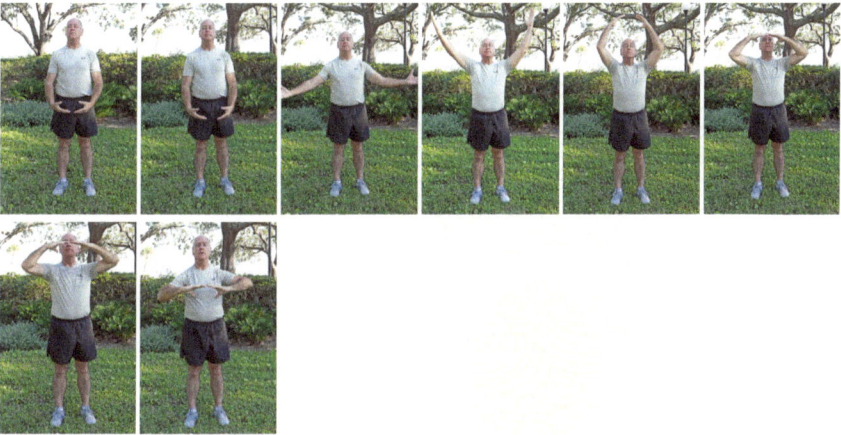

cleansing

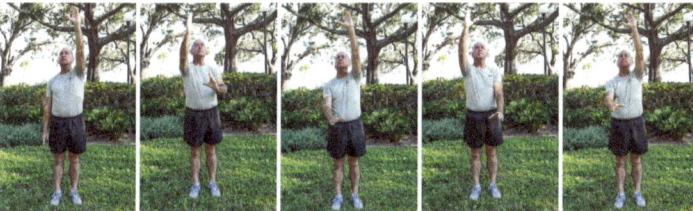

picking fruit

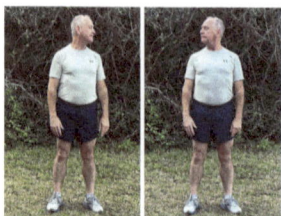

head turning - left & right

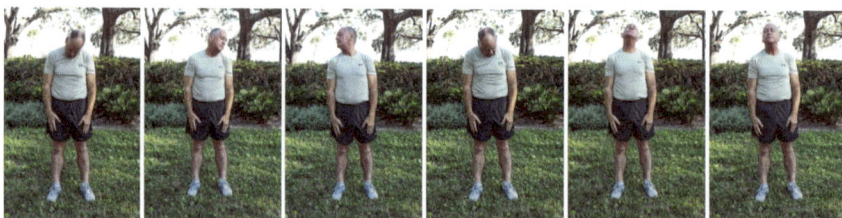

head circle

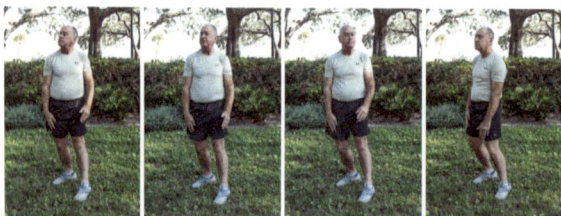

shoulders left side

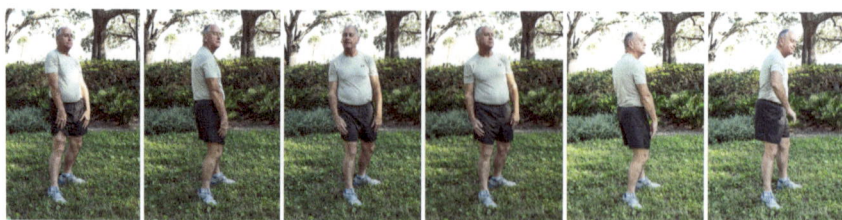

shoulders right side

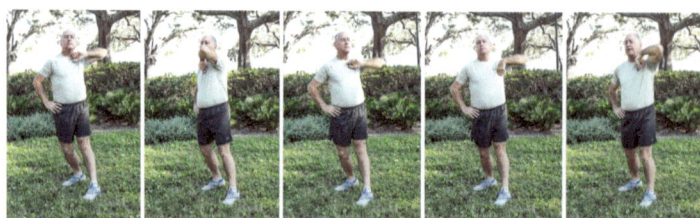

elbows left side

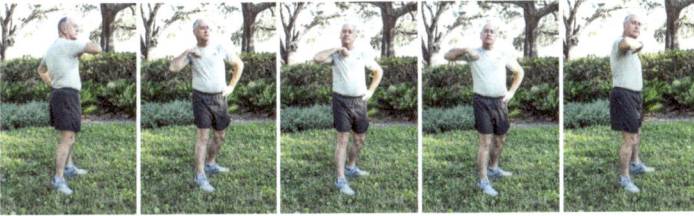

elbows right side

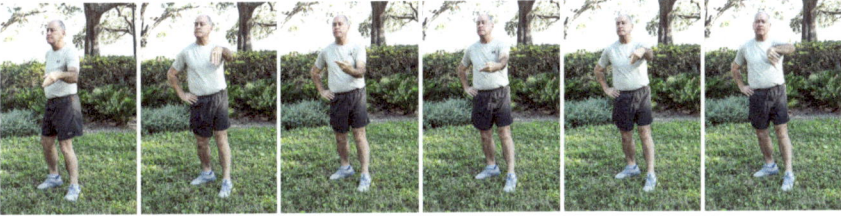

wrists - single left side

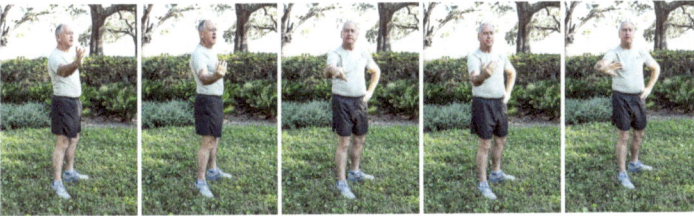

wrists - single right side

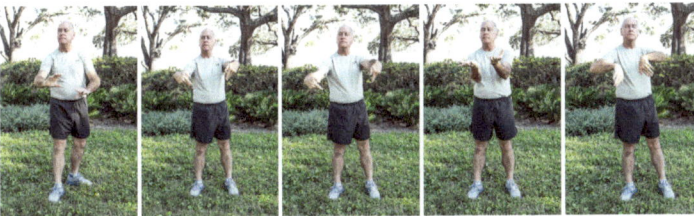

wrist - doubles

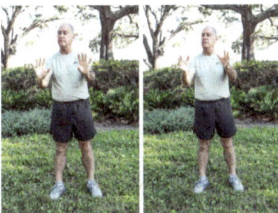

shake or stir the chi

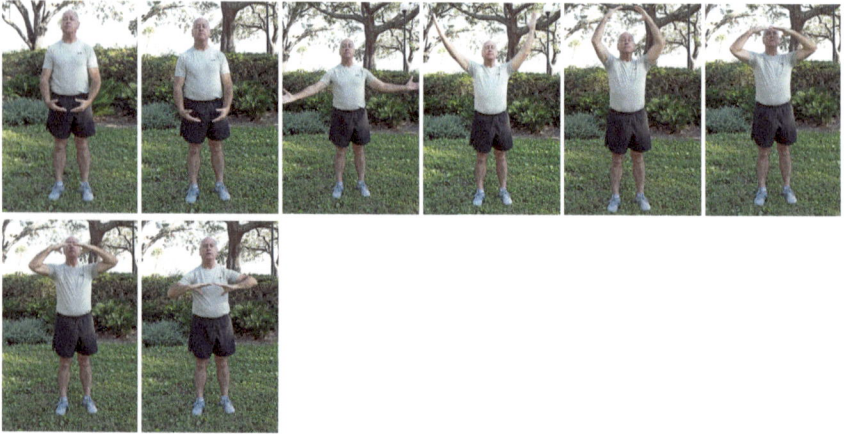

cleansing

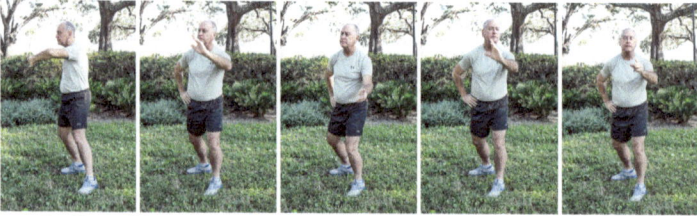

ward off & roll back left side

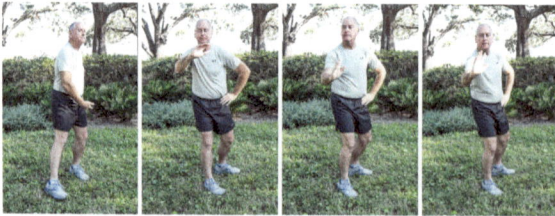

ward off & roll back - right side

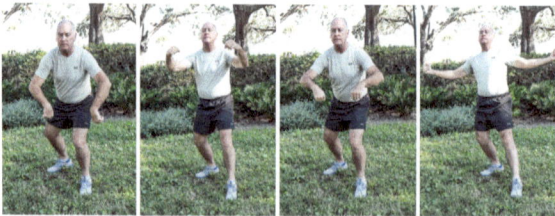

bend forward & pull back, open & close - left side

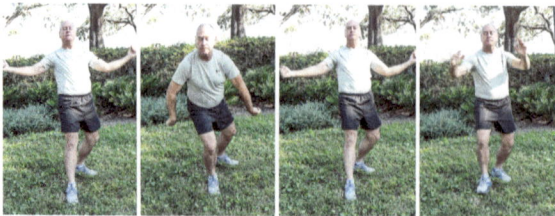

bend forward & pull back, open & close - right side

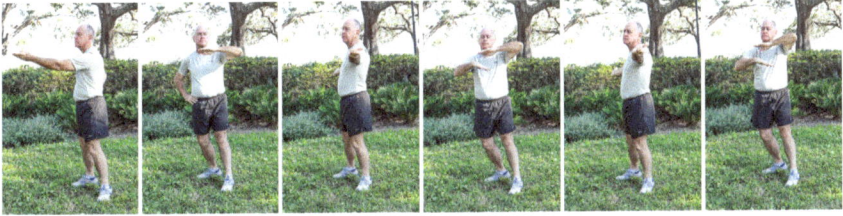

horizontal circle - single arm left side   horizontal circle - doubles left side

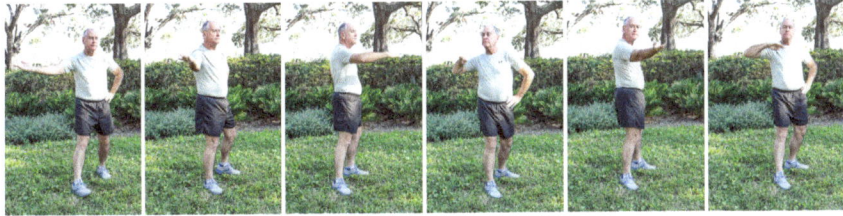

horizontal circle - single arm right side

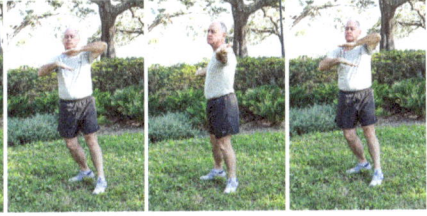

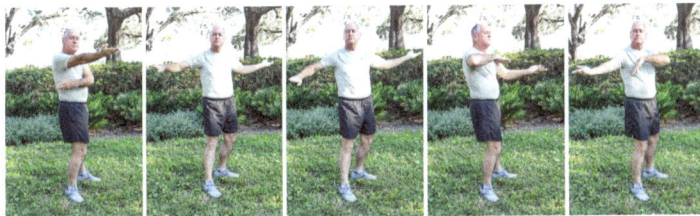

horizontal circle - doubles right side

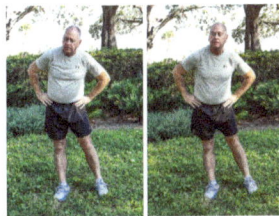

hips

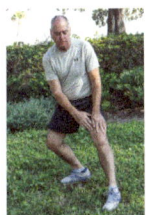

left knee -
outside circle

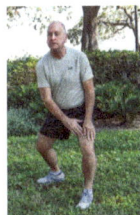

left knee -
inside circle

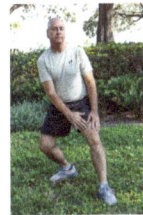

left knee -
forward & back

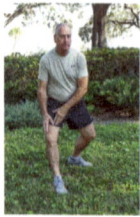

right knee - outside circle

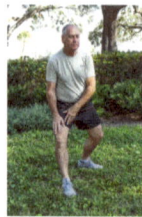

right knee - inside circle

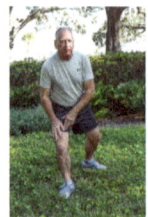

right knee - forward & back

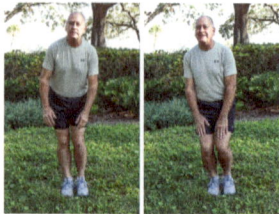

knees together

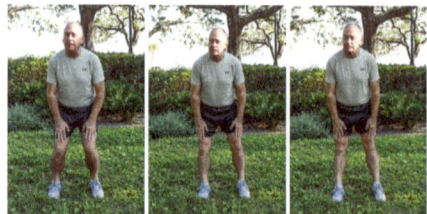

knees apart

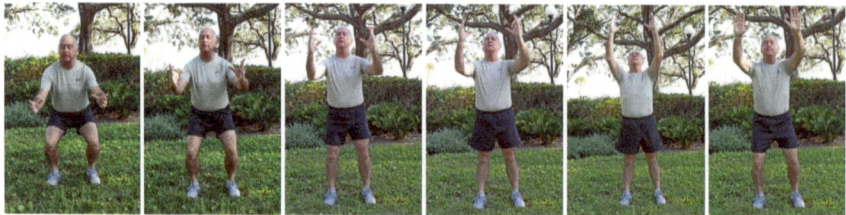

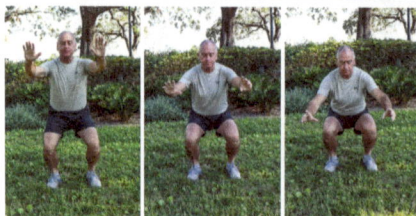

pick up ball lifting while holding the ball & circles

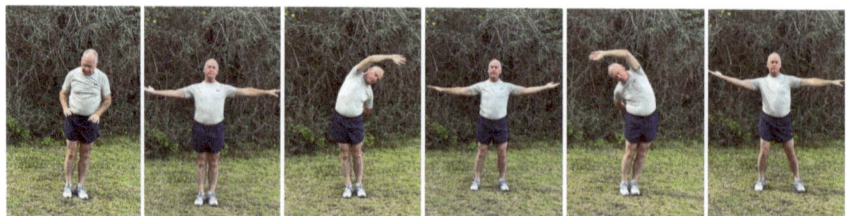

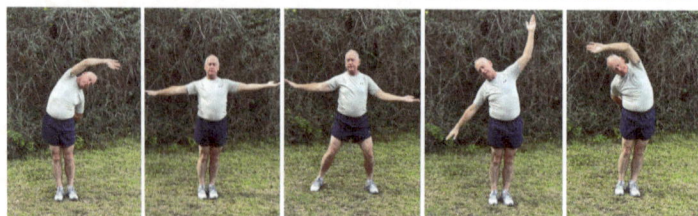

side tilt

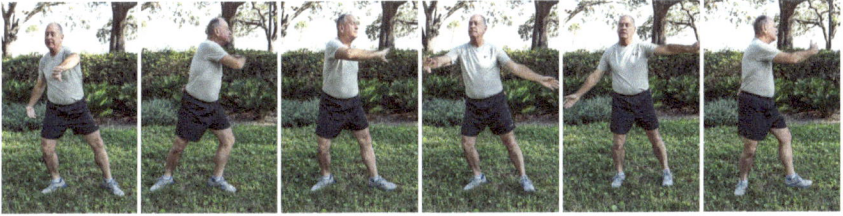

pat shoulder

elbow to toe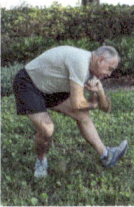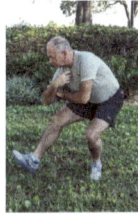

left side   right side

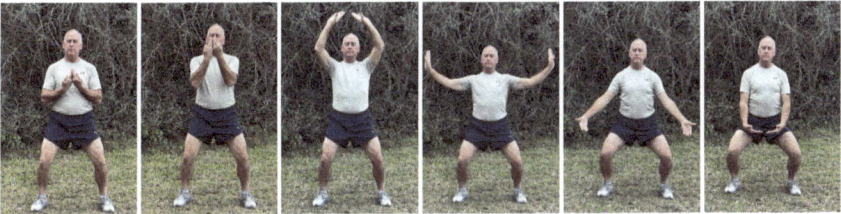

polish the mirror - outside circle

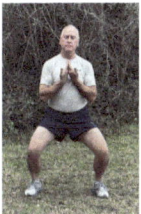

reverse direction

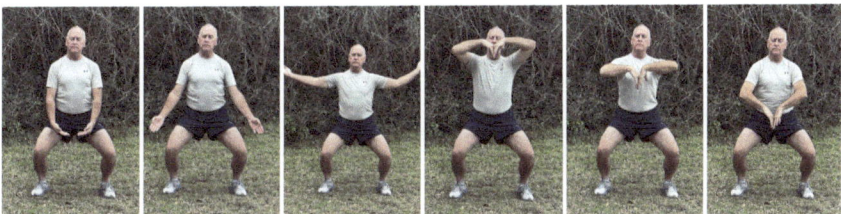

polish the mirror - inside circle

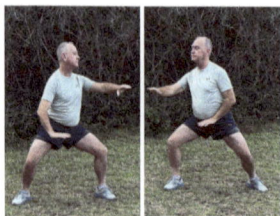

grind corn

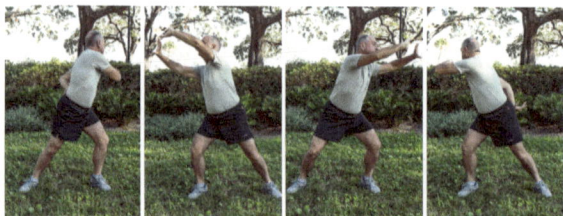

circle and look over shoulder

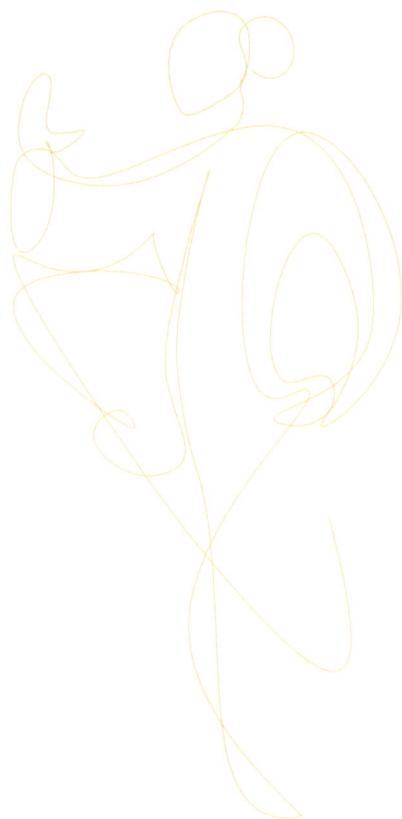

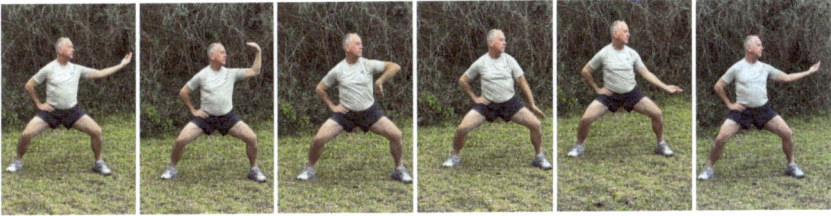

snake arm - left arm

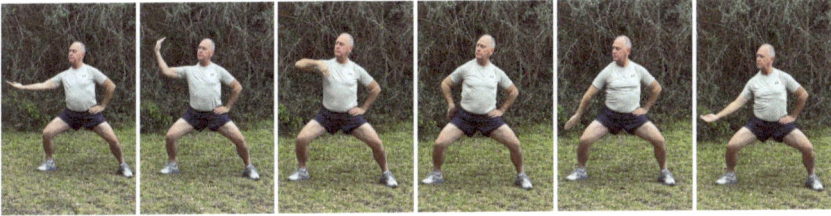

snake arm - right arm

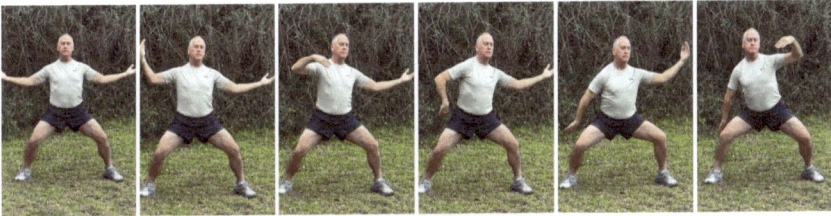

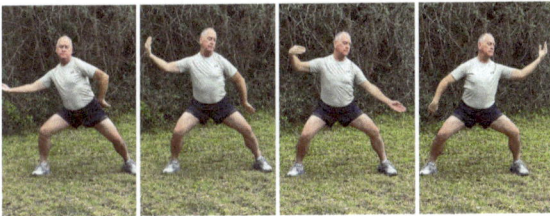

snake arm - doubles

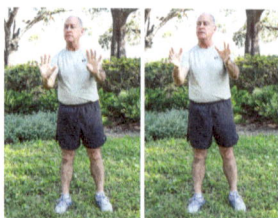

shake or stir the chi

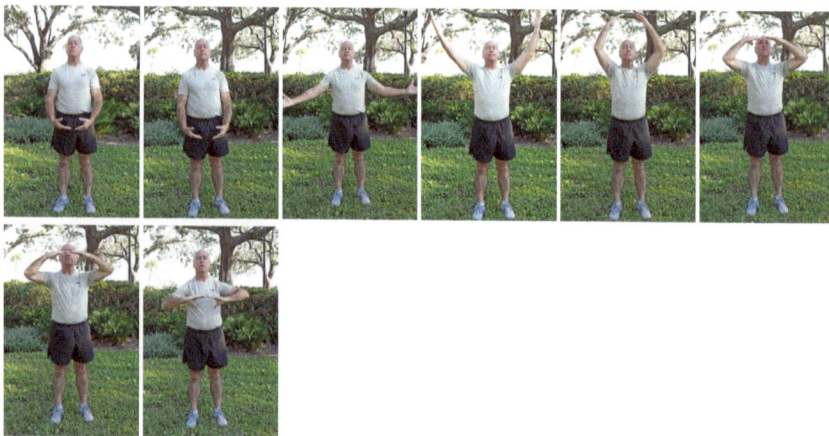

cleansing

3 STANDING MEDITATION POSTURES:

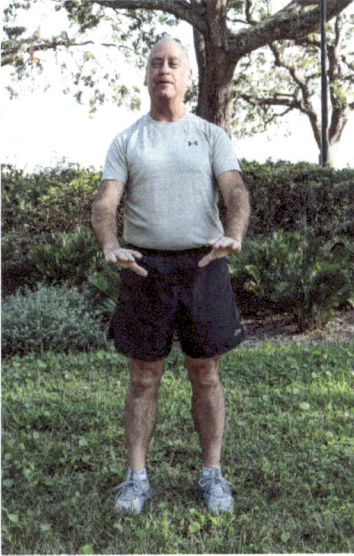

earth – posture

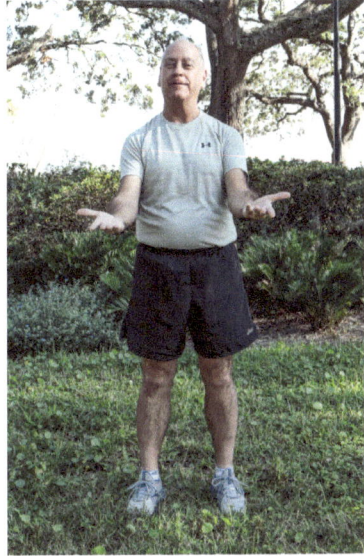

sky - heaven posture

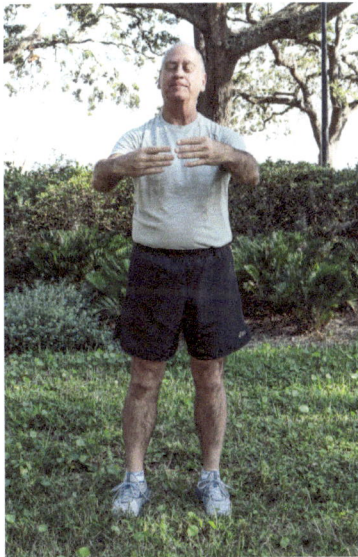

human - embrace posture

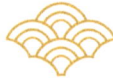

Cleansing	NEUTRAL STANCE	1-3 times
Picking Fruit		4-8 times
Head Turning		left & right 4-8 times
Head Circle		counterclockwise 4-8 times, then clockwise 4-8 times
Shoulders	LEFT SIDE FORWARD STANCE THEN SWITCH TO RIGHT SIDE FORWARD STANCE	**left side** - outside circle, rotate counterclockwise 4-8 times, then reverse rotation to inside circle, rotate clockwise
Elbows		**right side** - outside circle, rotate clockwise 4-8 times, then reverse rotation to inside circle, rotate counterclockwise
Wrists (Single)		
Wrists (Doubles)	NEUTRAL STANCE	Both Wrists Simultaneously **outside circles** (both hands simultaneously) 4-8 times reverse rotation to **inside circles** (both hands simultaneously) 4-8 times
Shake or Stir the Chi		Do an amount that feels right to you turning both wrists like turning a doorknob maintaining looseness as rapidly as possible
Cleansing		1-3 times

Ward off & roll back	**LEFT SIDE FORWARD STANCE**	• Left side forward 4-8 times • Right side forward 4-8 times
Bend forward & pull back	THEN SWITCH TO	
Horizontal Circle (Single & Doubles)	**RIGHT SIDE FORWARD STANCE**	
Hips	**NEUTRAL STANCE**	counterclockwise 4-8 times, then clockwise 4-8 times
Knees Individually	**LEFT SIDE** THEN SWITCH TO **RIGHT SIDE**	**outside circles** - 4-8 times **inside circles** - 4-8 times **forward & back** - 4-8 times
Knees Together	**NEUTRAL STANCE**	counterclockwise 4-8 times, then clockwise 4-8 times
Knees Apart		
Pick Up Ball	**NEUTRAL STANCE**	Up and Down 4-8 times
Lifting While Holding The Ball & Circles		counterclockwise 4-8 times, then clockwise 4-8 times
Side Tilt		stepping from side to side left and right side to side

Pat Shoulder	**HORSE STANCE** OR **NEUTRAL STANCE**	Shift weight onto the (R) foot, lift the (L) toes, pivot on the (L) heel, while turning from the waist, then press the (L) toes into the ground. Place the (L) hand behind the back and pat shoulder with your (R) hand. Repeat on the opposite side, alternating weight and ensure that when lowering the (R) toes the entire (R) foot presses into the ground with the (R) knee slightly forward.
Elbow to Toe	**NEUTRAL STANCE**	Stand, neutral, feet shoulder with apart, shift your weight to the (R). Pivot on your (L) heel, turning your waist (L), fold your arms with the (R) hand inside the (L) elbow, bend at the waist to aim your (L) elbow toward your (L) toes. Return to neutral, shift weight to the (L), repeat the movement to the (R). Hold each side for a count 4–8.
Polish The Mirror		Move hands back-to-back, lowering them in front of the body. Part hands at the bottom, extend arms to the sides with palms up, then raise them in a wide circle to meet at the top. Repeat this motion 4-8 times.
Grind Corn	**HORSE STANCE**	Begin in a Horse Stance, both palms facing down in front of the body, waist high. Start with the (R) hand circling to the (R) then the (L) hand circles to the (L). The (R) hand does an outside circle clockwise. The (L) hand does an outside circle counterclockwise. Alternating both hands were one leads than the other followers. It will create an infinity symbol or a figure 8.

Look Over Shoulder	**HORSE STANCE**	Begin in a Horse Stance with fingertips pointing toward each other, palms down in front of the body. As the waist turns (L), both hands rise to form a vertical circle, palms are up at the top, then lower and cross in front, with the (L) hand moving behind the back with palm facing out, and the (R) palm pressing away from the (L) shoulder. Root through your (L) foot, turn your waist, and look over your (L) shoulder. Reverse the circle by turning from the waist to the (R), both hands return to fingertips pointing towards each other palms down rise to form a vertical circle, palms are up at the top, then lower and cross in front, with the (R) hand moving behind the back with palm facing out, and the (L) palm pressing away from the (R) shoulder. Root through your (R) foot, turn your waist, and look over your (R) shoulder.
Shake Or Stir The Chi	**NEUTRAL STANCE**	Begin in a Neutral Stance, feet rooted, and cleanse by catching the Chi in front of the body. Shake loosely closed fists in an embrace position, turning from the waist with a forward and backward motion, or roll forearms with knuckles aligned in front. Relax arms to your sides, then inhale to raise them overhead in a "Y" shape, palms covering the crown, and exhale as hands lower, shifting back into a neutral stance.
Cleansing		

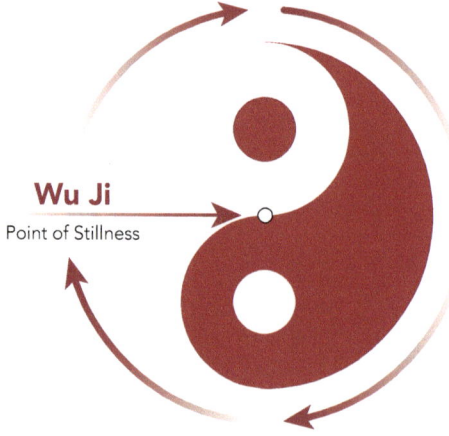

Wu Ji
Point of Stillness

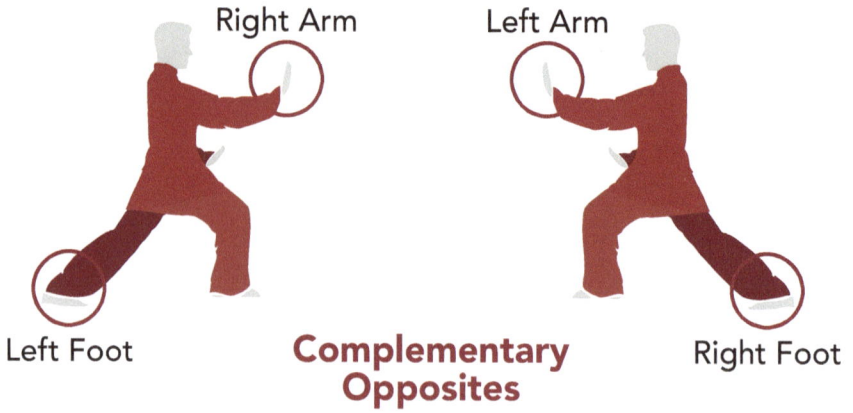

Right Arm

Left Arm

Left Foot

**Complementary
Opposites**

Right Foot

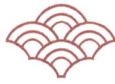

PART 3
Now is time to begin the Silk Reeling Qigong Routine

The beginning or opening movement is a cleansing hand motion.

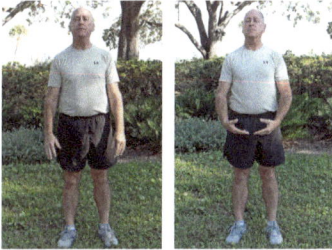

Wu Ji or Wu Chi

Begin by standing in a natural posture, a Neutral Stance (Wu Ji). Stand upright with the crown of your head to the sky, as if someone had a string pulling it gently upward. While doing this, keep your knees slightly bent and place your feet about shoulder-width apart, and rest your hands at the sides of your legs. Chin up and level. With your hands beside your body, from this naturally relaxed lower position, begin to raise the arms with palms cupped up together fingertips pointing towards each other.

Cleansing

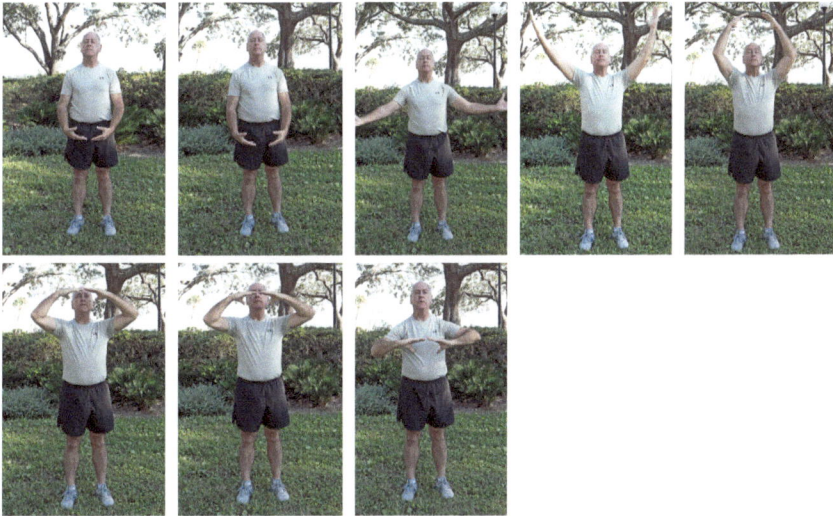

While doing this you want to be inhaling through your nose as you raise your arms fully extended from the side of the body allowing them to point to the sky like a funnel. Continuing this motion to over the head position. Make the hands come together forming a cup to cover the crown of the head with the palms facing down, fingers pointing at each other but do not touch.

During this exercise, the tongue is up, behind the teeth but not touching teeth like saying the letter L.

When we are covering the crown of the head and the palms down, slowly lower hands in front of body, fingers close but apart. As hands pass in front of the upper palate, lower the tongue from the roof of the mouth and exhale through the nose with the mouth closed. Exhaling, continue pressing downward with palms until arms are fully extended to lower the position with hands settling at the sides.

Repeat 3 times, or as many as you want to do.

Remember to breathe through the nose, inhale up, keep the tongue to the roof of the mouth and exhale down and out through the nose and at this point the tongue is lowered inside the mouth. Upon the start of the next cleansing, the tongue returns and is put back to the roof of the mouth for the remainder of the exercises.

This cleansing movement is a preparation for yourself and intended to clear the mind and relax peacefully, aware of yourself and surroundings.

Maintain mental focus and intention on the lower dan tien.

Remember that ideally all movement begins first from the lower dan tien, then extends to the rest of the body through fingertips, toes, and top of the head.

Inhale the breath, bringing the arms up allowing the fingertips to point directly up towards the sky like a funnel. The body with extended arms forms a Y in shape. The hands come back towards each other creating a cup covering the crown of the head. When the palms pass in front of the face, lower the tongue inside the mouth as you exhale down. Then, the tongue returns to the roof of the mouth. Shifting weight and continuing with the next exercise.

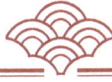

A Quick Overview

Left foot pressing down as the Right hand reaches upward

Right foot pressing down as the Left hand reaches upward

This connection is created by the internal
spiral turning beginning from the waist

Head Turning looking left & right and head circle rotation

Picking Fruit

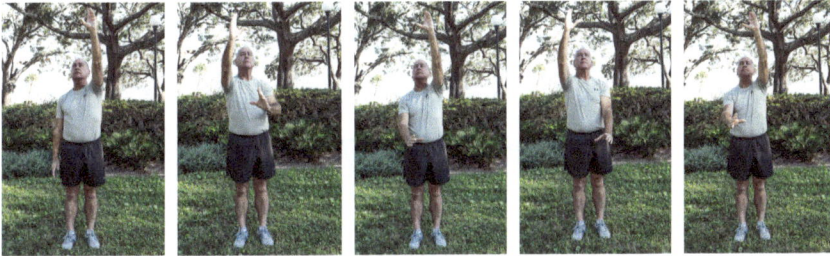

Begin from a Neutral Stance and the heels together with the feet slightly apart, we begin by alternating sides, reaching up as though picking fruit from a tree. Remember to always keep a slight bend in the elbow instead of letting the elbow lock, allowing for a natural extension of the arms. Repeat 8 times. Settle with a relaxing pause with arms resting down at sides of the legs.

If you can or are able, put your feet together as you are reaching up. The (L) foot is grounded or rooted by pressing down the weight into the earth or floor as the (R) hand goes up to grasp and picks the imaginary fruit just above the head.

In this exercise, (L) foot presses into the floor or ground and rooting while the (R) hand is rising. And (R) foot presses into the floor or ground and rooting while the (L) hand is rising.

Head Turning: Left & Right, and Head Circles

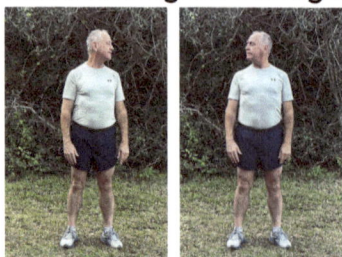

head turning - left & right

Begin from a Neutral Stance with the feet about shoulder width apart and arms resting down at sides. Slowly look to the left, then to the right, 4 times. Keep the spine aligned, upright, with the crown of the head up to the sky. Continuing, move head gently chin down towards the body circle to the left continuing the direction 4 times or 4 circle rotations. Reverse the direction of the circle rotation to the right. Complete the head circle 4 times or rotations.

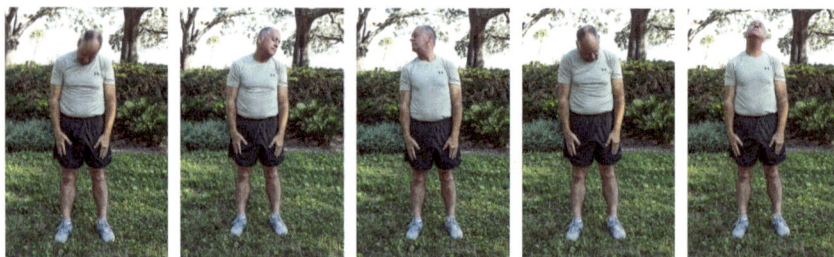

head circle

If you are turning the waist, it should happen on its own. What would seem like a simple exercise of just turning your head to look to the left with the neck exercise as you are rooting through your (R) foot pressing into the ground or floor to look to the left side, and then as you are rooting through your (L) foot to look right. There is a grounding or a rooting into the earth so that you maintain a good connection.

Shoulders

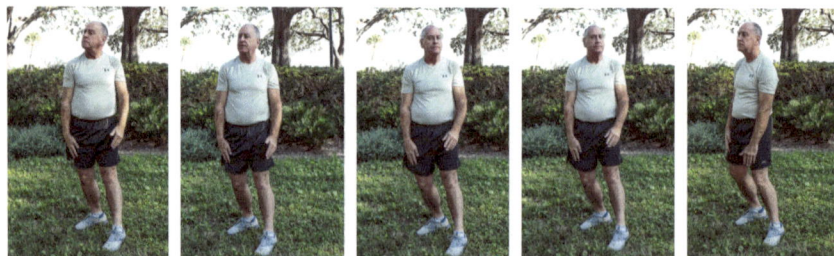

shoulders - left side

Begin with the (L) foot forward and the (R) foot back with the toes of the (L) foot pointed towards the right slightly less than 90 degrees with the hands resting at sides. As the waist turns, from the dan tien, the left shoulder moves forward, up, back, and down in an outside circle rotation. This is coming from the inside going towards the outside range (counterclockwise). Do this rotation 8 times. The (L) hand lightly traces a circle on the left thigh.

Reverse the rotational direction with figure 8 and lift shoulder at back, move forward, down, back, and up in an inside circle rotation from outside to inside (clockwise). Do this rotation 8 times.

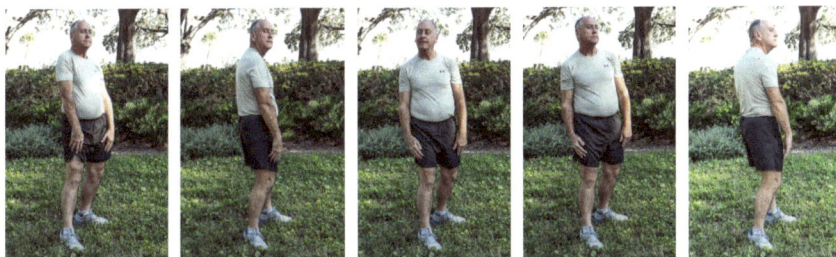

shoulders - right side

Changing position by reversing feet. Place the (R) foot forward and the (L) foot back with the toes of the (R) foot pointed towards the left slightly less than 90 degrees with the hands resting at the sides. Continue to repeat the shoulder rotation movement on the right side (clockwise). Focus on the use of the waist creating a figure 8 motion as the origin of the shoulder's rotation.

Reverse the rotational direction with figure 8 and lift shoulder at back, move forward, down, back, and up in circle rotation from inside to outside (counterclockwise). Do this rotation 8 times. On the shoulder exercise, you are making a circle.

It is like you are drawing a circle with your shoulder. As I am lifting, I am always beginning from the bottom. Points are turning the waist right to go left. Then as I am lifting, I am rooting through my (R) foot, pressing into the ground or floor. Then when you reverse, the same thing goes on. You are initiating everything from the waist to create the circle that is coming through in the shoulder.

So, I am not just turning. I am just not rolling my shoulder. That is simply a superficial way of doing it. I am rolling through my entire body, turning from the waist down and reversing. And for comfort, you can make a circle on the front leg with your hand on the same side of the body, if that helps get the rotation of the shoulder. The (L) hand can be on the left thigh or the (R) hand on the right thigh as comfortable.

Elbows

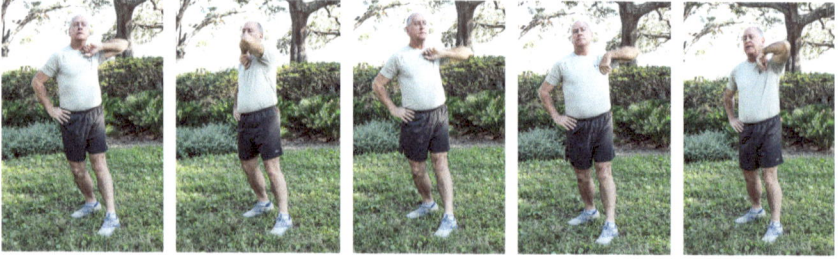

elbows - left side

Begin with your (L) foot forward and (R) foot back as in the shoulders exercise with (R) hand on hip.

With your left fingers form a loosely closed fist, lightly touching the chest. As the waist turns, the left elbow moves forward, up, back, and down in a circle from the inside to rotate to the outside 8 times (clockwise). Left fist traces a circle on the chest.

Reverse rotational direction with figure 8 and lift elbow at back, move forward, down, back, and up in a circle from the outside to the inside 8 times (counterclockwise).

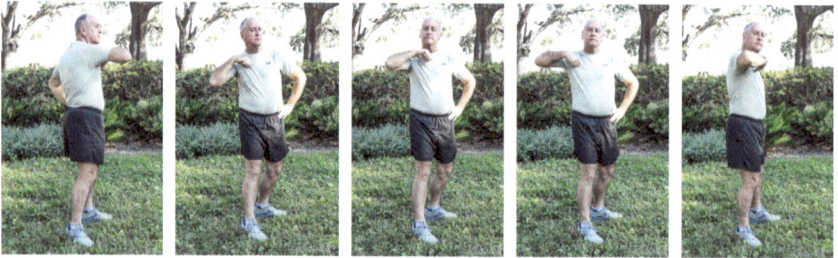

elbows - right side

Reverse feet, repeat the elbow movement on the right side. Maintain focus on the use of hip and waist creating a figure 8 motion as origin of elbow movement.

Reverse rotational direction with figure 8 and lift elbow at back, move forward, down, back, and up in a circle from the outside to the inside 8 times (clockwise).

The palm of the hand not doing the exercise should be on the waist or the hip of the other side of the body. And then if you are able, gently form a fist and you are circling on the chest. If able to make that connection, it is like drawing a circle with the point tip of the elbow. And again, you want to root or ground through the feet with the top of the head extended, some rooting from the right side to turn the waist, rooting for the left side to come back.

On this exercise that there's circling. It is like drawing a circle with the elbow. But again, it is not just circling the elbow, it is turning from the waist, from inside the body to the outside in a clockwise rotation.

You should feel like a figure 8 taking place within the feet by the turning of the waist. At the same time, we draw a circle with the tip of the elbow.

Wrist

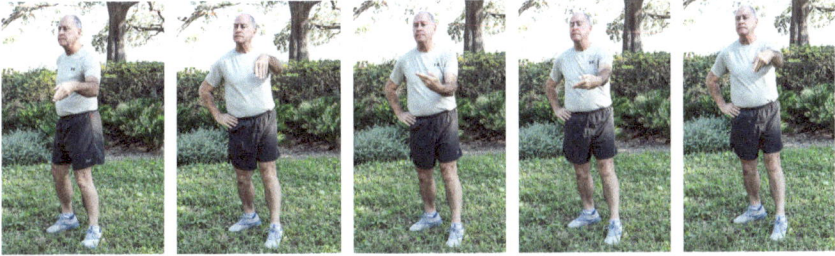

wrist - single left side

Begin with the (L) foot forward and the (R) foot back with the (R) hand on the right hip. With my left arm extended and my elbow slightly bent. As the waist turns, the wrist turns like a doorknob in a counterclockwise motion 8 times in an outside circle directional rotation. Then, reverse the rotational direction 8 times inside circle direction (counterclockwise). Reverse feet, repeat with right wrist 8 times in each rotational direction.

Initially it is like you are rolling your palm around a doorknob. Here I am doing what I call an outside circle. Because it is on my (L)hand. It is a counterclockwise motion. But for convenience, it is easier to just say, do an outside circle. Moving away from the torso, away from the body.

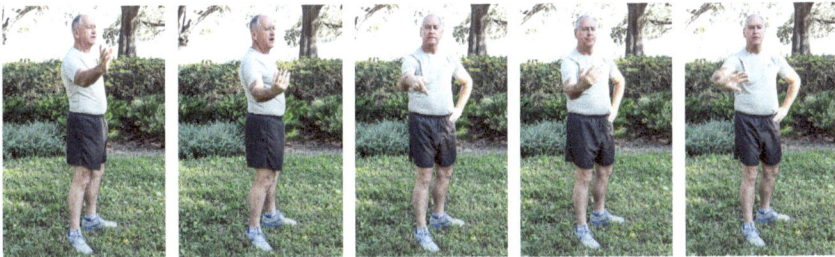

wrist - single right side

And then you can reverse. It is an inside circle again. It comes towards the body and from the ground this time, turning the way so that there is a connection through the feet. Rolling your wrist around the door.

Here you can keep the spinal column aligned, lifting the crown of the head again, so that there is grounding through the feet.

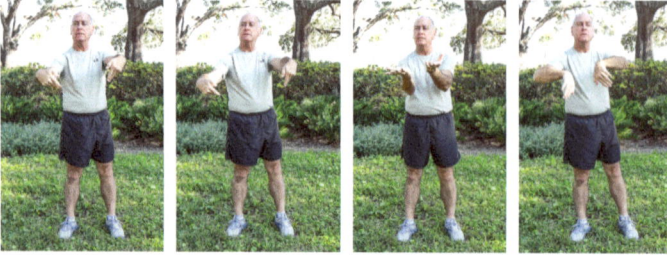

wrists - doubles

Begin in a Neutral Stance, with the feet shoulder-width apart, extend both arms forward in front of the body, remembering the elbows are extended yet not locking at joints. As the waist turns, move both wrists inside to outside circular rotations 8 times; Reverse the rotational direction to move outside to inside 8 times.

Shake or Stir the Chi

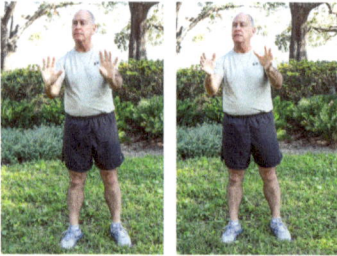

Begin in a Neutral Stance, with arms extended forward in front of the body, loosely shake both wrists in front of the body.
You want to twist the wrists and shake the chi in the palms. Turn the wrists. Loosening and relaxing let the arms go back down to the sides of the body.

Cleansing

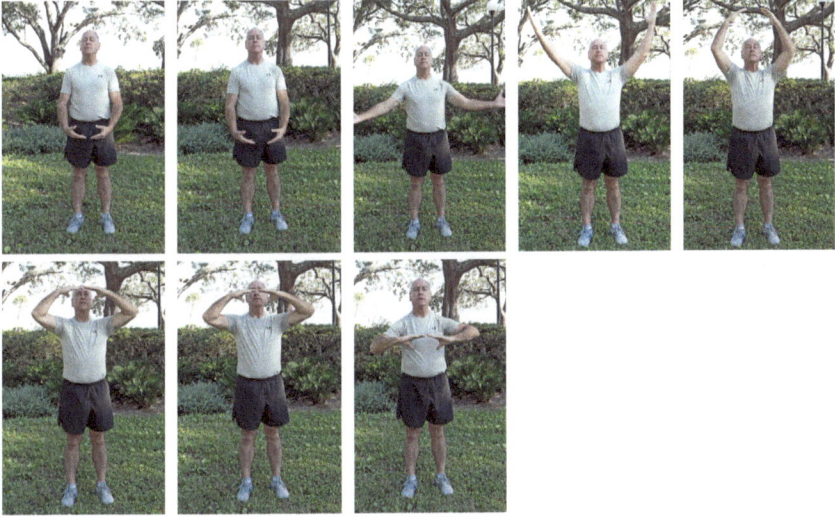

Repeat the opening movement and read that section again.

Beginning the cleansing exercise by inhaling the breath bringing the arms up, allowing the fingertips to point directly up towards the sky like a funnel Body forms a Y in shape, the hands come back towards each other creating a covering over the crown of the head. When the palms pass in front of the face, lower the tongue inside the mouth. As you exhale down. Then, the tongue returns to the roof of the mouth. Shifting weight to begin the next exercise.

Ward Off & Roll Back

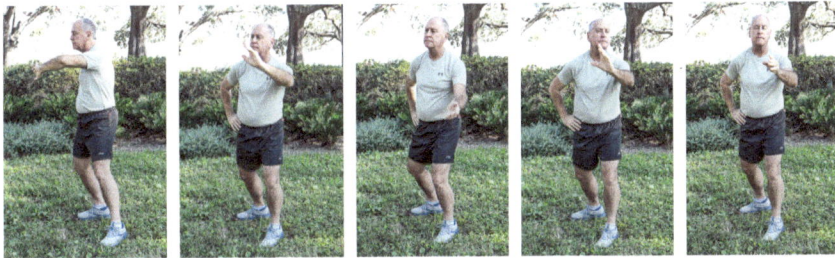

left side

Begin with the (L) foot forward, (R) foot back, (R) hand on hip; As waist turns from dan tien, (L) hand, palm up, moves or flows down, then cross body in circle to scoop up water. When fully extended, the arm draws back and out with the palm down completing the circle beside the body. Repeat smoothly 8 times. Reverse feet and hands and repeat with the right side.

Be sure to keep the connection that you root through the rear foot grounding to go forward.

Turning from the waist. You want to stay connected as you make the transition. Again, root from the rear foot to go forward. Rooting into the ground from the forward foot to go back.

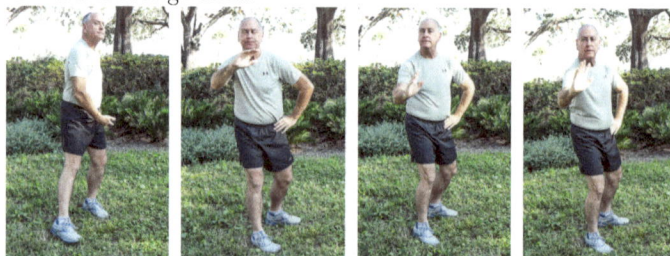

right side

Bend Forward & Pull Back Open & Close

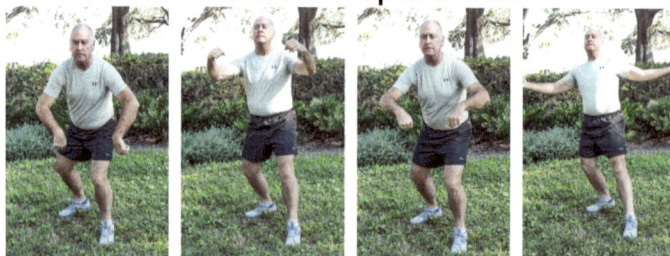

left side

Begin with the (L) foot forward, (R) foot back, hands form loose fist; elbows not locked, arms extended to each side and head up; Begin by moving forward from the abdomen, waist, dan tien and then moving or going backwards. Use your legs to move forward. Lean back, opening the chest area by pulling back, then bend forward bringing fists down and back at the sides, closing. Continue by bringing fists up and out to sides, opening the chest area pulling and leaning back slightly. Head remains up so eyes can see the horizon throughout forward and backward motion. Breathe from dan tien. Repeat 8 times.

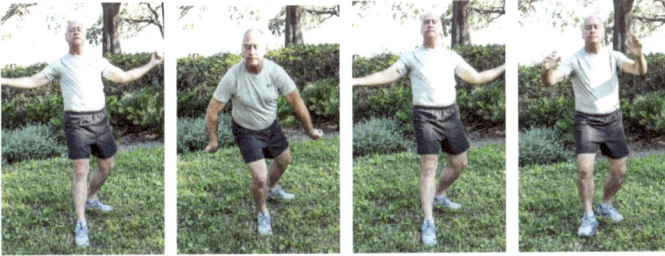

right side

Reverse the feet position to (R) foot forward and (L) foot back. Repeat 8 times with the (R) foot forward.

When you are bending forward, pay attention to the rear foot heel that stays down pressing into the ground for connection or rooting to the earth.

REMINDER: *pay attention to the fact that you are rooting through the rear foot to go forward, keeping the rear heel down.*

Horizontal Circle

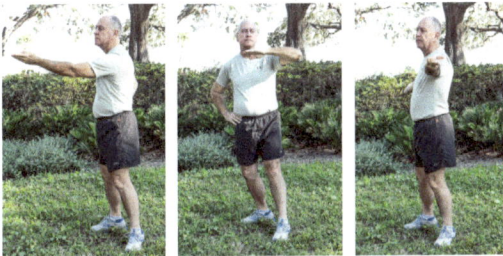

horizontal circle - single arm left side

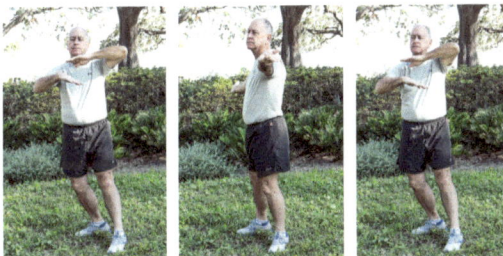

horizontal circle - doubles left side

Begin with your (L) foot forward and your (R) foot back and your (R) hand on your right-side hip; As your waist turns, keeping your left arm at chest level elbow not locked extended forward. (L) hand, palm up with thumb tucked, moves. across in front of the body from left to right. Focusing on dan tien, movement comes from turning the waist. (L) turning (L) palm down, (L) draw (L) hand back in front of head at chin level to beginning point. Repeat 8 times.

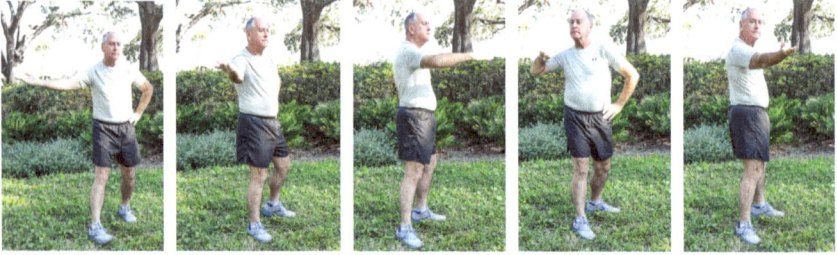

horizontal circle - single arm right side

Reverse feet and repeat with right side 8 times. (Focus: on use of hip motion in a horizontal figure 8)

🏵 REMINDER: *pay attention to the fact that you are pressing and rooting through the rear foot to go forward and keep the rear heel down.*

This is called a horizontal circle. Palms up. Come to the front of the body and turn away from the palms down, maintaining a horizontal line in front of the body. Relaxing the upper body. Turning from the waist.

🏵 REMINDER: *pay attention to the changing of your weight through the feet as well, so that the feet stay firmly rooted.*

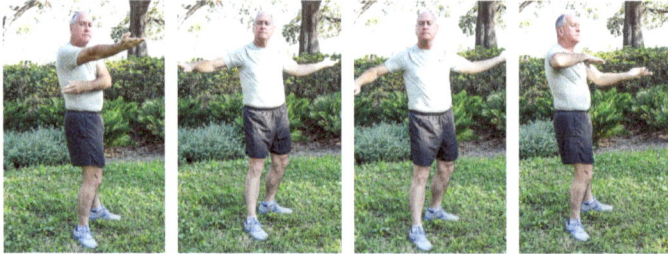

horizontal circle - doubles right side

This is an option that is a more advanced technique based on Horizontal Circle, Single Arm. The exercise is done the same way except the other arm (not the leading side) is added into the sequence by tucking that palm hand down and under the horizontal arm, then turning the palm up as it moves backwards horizontally away such that at full extension both palms are facing up and arms fully extended (not locked) before continuing the next count of the range of motion.

Hips - Waist

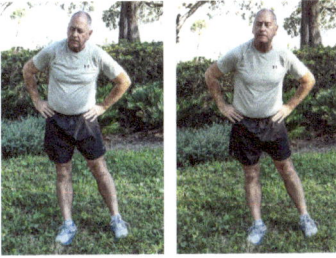

circle right & circle left

Begin in a Neutral Stance, head up, knees not locked, feet shoulder width apart, and my hands are on my hips; Move hips in a horizontal circle clockwise, starting from left, hips move forward, right, back, and left, 8 times. Reverse direction counterclockwise with a figure 8 and repeat 8 times from right to left. Circling from the waist. Relaxing the upper body. Turning from the waist.

Knees individually

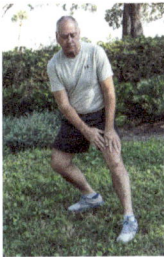

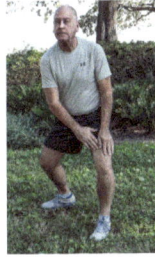

| left knee - outside circle | left knee - inside circle | left knee - forward & back |

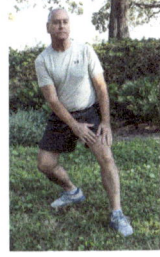

Keeping both feet flat to the ground, (L) foot forward, (R) foot back, knees not locked, both hands can be lightly touching or rest on the left thigh. This can also be for protection of alignment. As the waist turns from the dan tien, the left knee moves right, forward, left, and back in a gentle circle. Repeat 8 times in to out. Reverse direction and repeat 8 times out to in with the left knee. Straightening (L) foot, shifting weight forward and back. Repeat 8 times. Reverse feet and repeat 8 times in to out and 8 times out to in with the right knee. Straightening the (R) foot, shifting weight forward and back. Repeat 8 times.

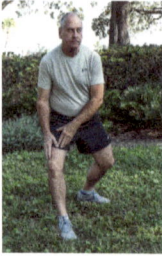

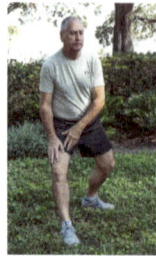

| right knee - outside circle | right knee - inside circle | right knee - forward & back |

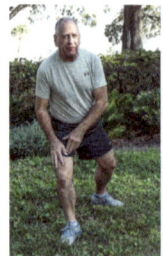

Here, you want to pay attention to the changing of the weight through the feet as well, so that the feet stay firmly rooted.

I tend to do a medium to a low stance. They were circling, but I was not hovering over. And I am bringing the weight back on to the rear foot or the rear leg. Create a circle.

Keep in mind that if you are in a higher stance, it does not take as far to go outside that range.

Knees together

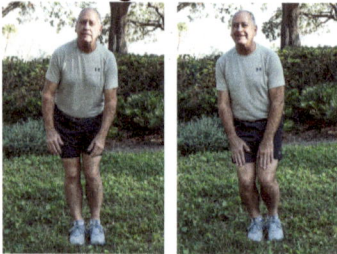

circle right, circle left

My hands are on top of my thighs, fingers lightly touching legs. Move knees in a circle 4 times from left to right; Reverse direction, right to left 4 times.

Bring your feet together. As close as you comfortably can. Circle them together to the right clockwise. Keep your feet completely flat to the ground as best as possible.

Reverse the direction of the circle. Circling to the left and counterclockwise. Stepping out into a neutral position.

Knees apart

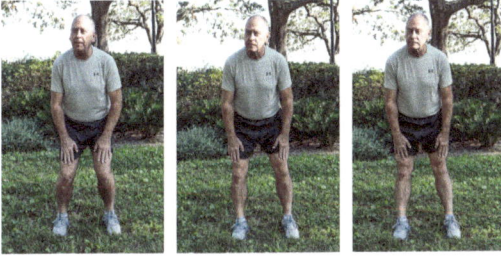

outside & inside circles

Repeat with knees apart 4 times in each direction; Knees apart, move knees in to out 4 times; Reverse and move knees out to in 4 times.

Outside circles. Smooth out any rough edges within the circle. And here we are going the reverse inside circle coming in towards the body. Feet are firmly planted to the ground.

Pick Up Ball

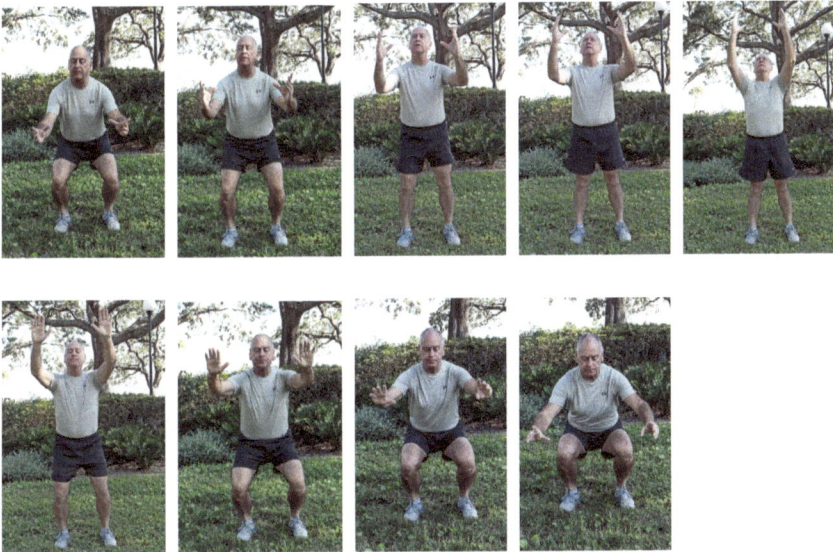

Begin in a Neutral Stance with the feet about shoulder width apart. Sink your energy in the chi, squat the body, and pick up (imaginary) ball, raise the ball in front of the body to overhead height. Palms down, lower ball. Palms face one another, fingertips point to the sky at the uppermost position of exercise. Repeat 8 times beginning with squats.

NOTE: for strength training, one could use a "medicine" leather ball or other weighted ball can be used.

Returning to the ground. Sink. Extend the fingertips to the sky. Again. Never lock your knees, keep a natural bend.

Be aware of the alignment of the spine. Through the crown of the head.

Holding the Ball (circles)
circle right & circle left

Begin in a Neutral Stance, feet apart; As the waist turns, lift the ball over head from left to right in front of body, bring down and across to the left to make a circle. Repeat 8 times. Reverse direction with a figure 8 and repeat 8 times. Keep spine aligned; top of head (crown) to sky.

Turning from the waist. Circling. Allow the waist to circle the arms.

Palms. Face one another. Be aware of the changing weight through the feet. Here we create a loop to return. Reverse the circle.

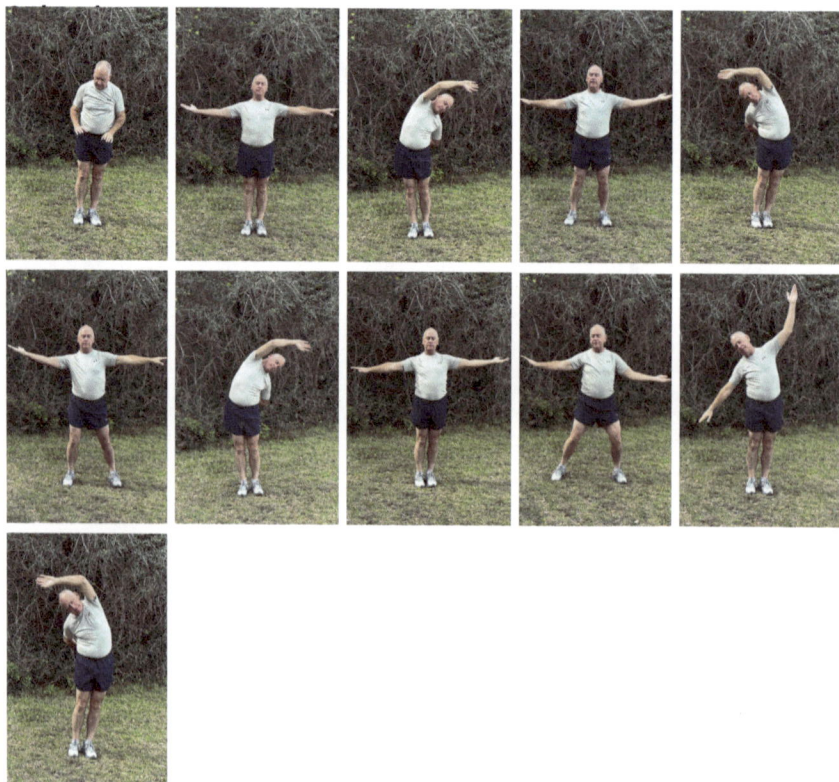

NOTE: *when doing the side tilts, you will always step left & bend right, pause for a moment with balanced control then continue with step right & bend left. pausing again for a moment with balanced control before stepping left and bending to the right side.*

Beginning in a Neutral Stance, feet apart, arms extended to the sides. Bring your (L) foot beside your (R) foot; (L) palm down, (R) palm up; Bend sideways at waist to the left. As the body bends the (L) hand moves down and behind the body, the (R) hand rises to an arc above the head. Reverse direction, step to the side with (L) foot. Bring your (R) foot beside your (L) foot, (L) palm up, (R) palm down; Bend sideways at waist to the right. As the body bends the (R) hand moves down and behind the body, and the (L) hand rises to arc above the head. Repeat 8 times.

Ideally, when doing the Side Tilt and the steps from side to side, you should have enough control that as you extend your foot to the side, that you could stop before putting any weight on it and retract the foot (leg) and bring it back to the position that you are. There should be enough control that you could stop before putting any weight on that foot completing the new side. Yet having the ability you could continue putting the full weight on the foot to make the transfer of weight to the other side. So, step lightly to the side, putting the full weight onto it when safely transitioned, then shift and do the stepping lightly before putting weight into the other side and transferring full weight back to the other side.

Pat Shoulder

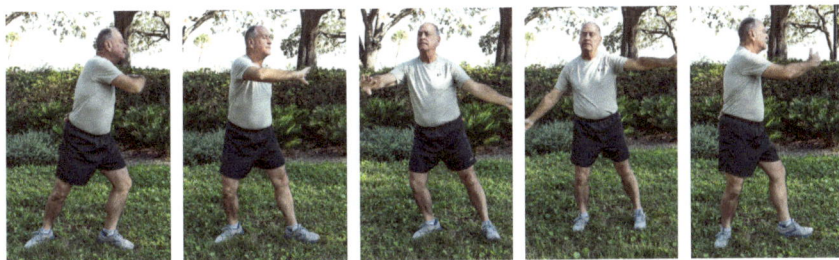

Begin in a Neutral Stance, facing front, feet shoulder width apart; arms are extended out at the sides. Shift weight onto the (R) foot, lift the (L) toes, pivot on the (L) heel, while turning from the waist to the (L), then press the (L) toes into the ground. The entire (L) foot is now pressing into the ground. My (L) knee moves forward slightly but never beyond the point above the toes.

The (L) hand moves down and behind the back, with the back of palm touching back, if possible, while the (R) hand moves in front of the body and pats (L) shoulder with your (R) hand. (R) foot remains flat, pointing in front.

By alternating the weight between the (L) and (R) sides, this ensures that when lowering the (L) toes the entire (L) foot presses into the ground with the (L) knee slightly forward

Reverse movement to go to the (R) side. Shift weight onto the (L) foot, lift the (R) toes, pivot on the (R) heel, while turning from the waist to the (R), then press the (R) toes into the ground. The entire (R) foot is now pressing into the ground. My (R) knee moves forward slightly but never beyond the point above the toes

By alternating the weight between the (L) and (R) sides, this ensures that when lowering the (R) toes the entire (R) foot presses into the ground with the (R) knee slightly forward.

Repeat 4-8 times.

Return to Neutral Stance or Horse Stance, both feet flat, facing front.

friendly reminder: after turning and adjusting the appropriate foot's toes, sometimes people will bring the rear heel up in motion. you do not want that. after completing the foot's toe lift and pivot, you want your foot to be firmly planted and pressing down which creates what i describe as "rooting".

Elbow to Toe

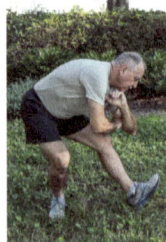
left

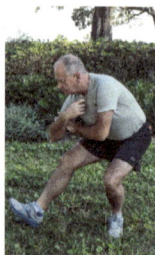
right

Begin in a Neutral Stance, facing front, feet shoulder width apart, As in Pat Shoulder, shift your weight to the (R) side. Lift (L) toes, pivot on your (L) heel. As the waist turns to the (L), fold your arms with the (R) hand inside the (L) elbow.

Bend at the waist and aim your (L) elbow toward your upturned (L) toes. You can keep your head and chin slightly up or lean towards the toes. Yet your weight must be sinking or sitting on your (R) leg for support, strength, and safety. The

(R) foot remains facing the front and the (R) knee is bent. Hold for a count of 8.

Begin in a Horse Stance, both palms facing down in front of the body, waist high.

Begin by turning from the waist to the (R), as the (R) hand begins circling to the (R), the (R) hand rises and circles slightly higher than the (L) hand.

Changing circle direction.

Now, the (L) hand circles to the (L), and the (L) hand rises and circles slightly higher than the (R) hand as the (R) hand lowers.

The (R) hand does an outside circle – clockwise. The (L) hand does an outside circle – counterclockwise. Alternating with both hands where one hand leads than the other hand follows. Then it changes so now the follower hand begins leading the direction, and the previous hand is now the follower. It will create an infinity symbol or a figure 8.

Reverse direction and as waist turn, a complete circle is repeated. The leading hand is always above the following hand.

There is an alternating weight shift between the feet as we alternate from the (R) hand lead circle then changing to the (L) hand lead circle and continuing back to the (R) hand starting a new lead cycle.

My (R) palm pressing down, rooting through the (R) foot to go left. We are adding to our (L) foot to continue circling back to the right-side weight.

My (L) palm pressing down, rooting through the (L) foot to go left. We are adding to our (R) foot to continue circling back to the left side weight.

Hold each side for a count 4–8.

Return to Neutral Stance or Horse Stance with both feet flat, facing front.

Polish the Mirror

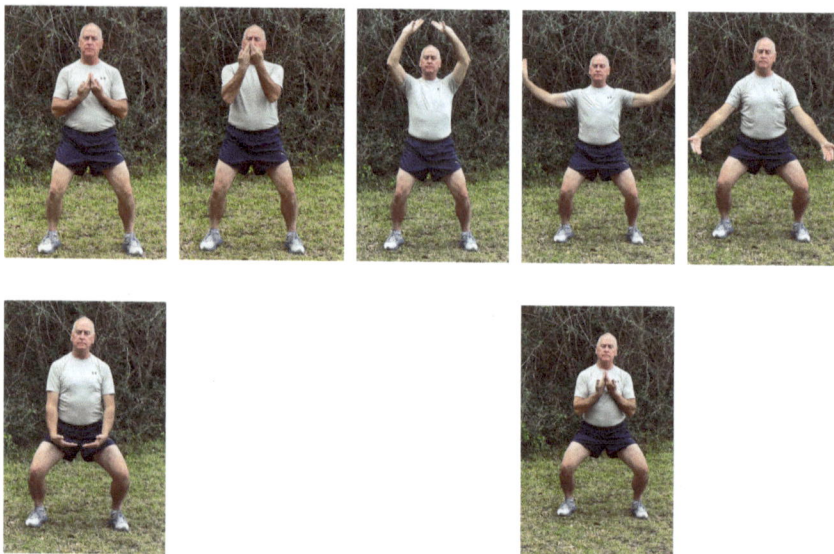

outside circle   reverse direction

Begin in a Horse Stance, hands move towards each other, fingertips leading, palms up, until fingers touch and backs of hands are together with knuckles nearly touching. Hands rise in front of the body, parting near the top of head. Palms press forward, away from the body, hands turning down, arms extend to each side as arms lower and come together again in front of the body. The left arm moves in a counterclockwise circle and the right arm in a clockwise circle. Repeat 4 times.

Once we are doing an inhale up. Exhale down the back of the palms. Come together. Using your legs you lift your palms apart. Keep your shoulders relaxed with the upper body. And the lower body comes together so that when I am lifting, ideally, the hands are rising as the legs are rising into the upper point. And then as we come down with the palm, our legs also come down.

Polish the Mirror - Inside Circle

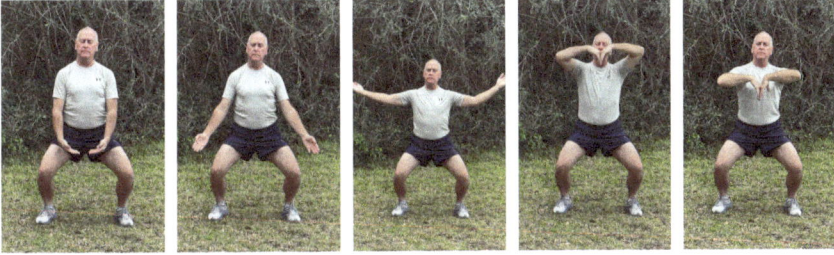

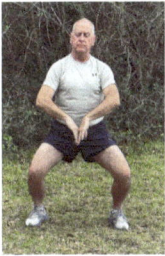

inside circle

Reverse the direction to begin an inside circle rotation. The back of the palms move parallel, lowering in front of the body. The hands part and separate at the bottom of the circle, arms extend to the sides, palms turn up. Hands rise in a wide circle to come together at the top of the circle. Back of the palms continue to come down in front of the body to repeat the circle rotation. Repeat 4 times.

Grind Corn

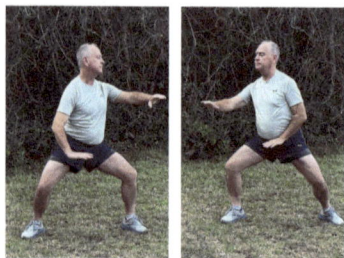

Begin in a Horse Stance, both palms facing down in front of the body, waist high.

Begin by turning from the waist to the (R), as the (R) hand begins circling to the (R), the (R) hand rises and circles slightly higher than the (L) hand.

Changing circle direction.

Now, the (L) hand circles to the (L), and the (L) hand rises and circles slightly higher than the (R) hand as the (R) hand lowers.

The (R) hand does an outside circle – clockwise. The (L) hand does an outside circle – counterclockwise. Alternating with both hands where one hand leads than the other hand follows. Then it changes so now the follower hand begins leading the direction, and the previous hand is now the follower. It will create an infinity symbol or a figure 8.

Reverse direction and as waist turn, a complete circle is repeated. The leading hand is always above the following hand.

There is an alternating weight shift between the feet as we alternate from the (R) hand lead circle then changing to the (L) hand lead circle and continuing back to the (R) hand starting a new lead cycle.

My (R) palm pressing down, rooting through the (R) foot to go left. We are adding to our (L) foot to continue circling back to the right-side weight. My (L) palm pressing down, rooting through the (L) foot to go left. We are adding to our (R) foot to continue circling back to the left side weight.

Look Over Shoulder

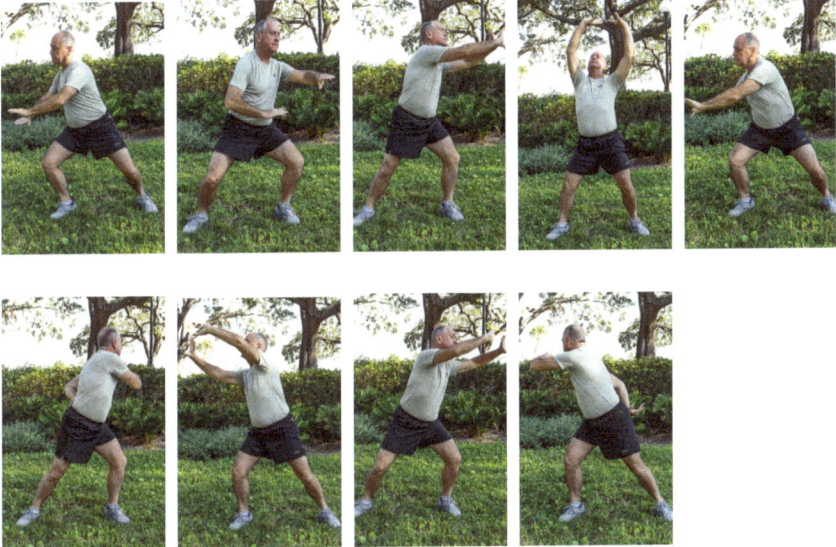

left side & right side

Begin in a Horse Stance with fingertips pointing toward each other, without touching, the palms face down in front of the body. As the waist turns (L), both hands rise to form a vertical circle, palms are up at the top, then hands lower and cross in front of the body,

the hands separate and part their near connection with the (L) hand moving behind the back with palm facing out, while the (R) palm presses away from the (L) shoulder. Root through your (L) foot, turn your waist, and look over your (L) shoulder.

Reverse the circle by turning from the waist to the (R), both hands return to fingertips pointing towards each other palms down rise to form a vertical circle, palms are up at the top, then lower and cross in front, with the (R) hand moving behind the back with palm facing out, and the (L) palm pressing away from the (R) shoulder. Root through your (R) foot, turn your waist, and look over your (R) shoulder.

Snake Arm

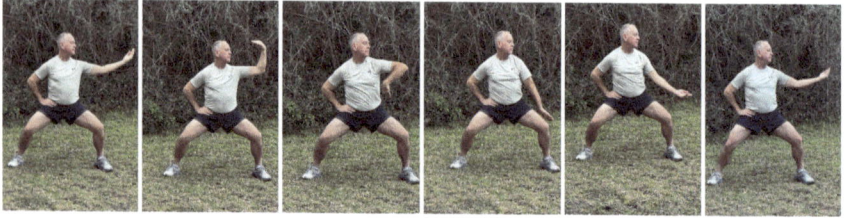

snake arm - left arm

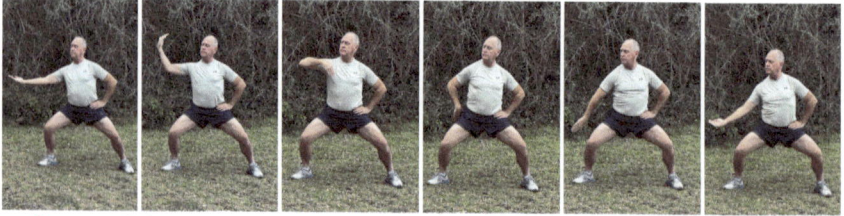

snake arm - right arm

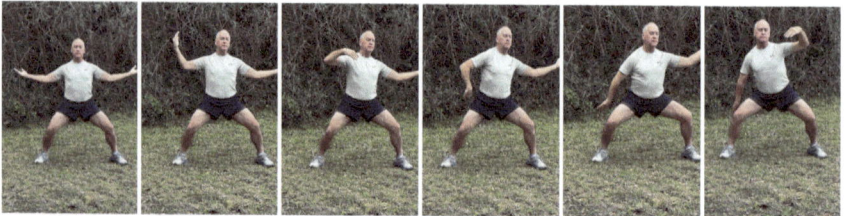

snake arm - doubles

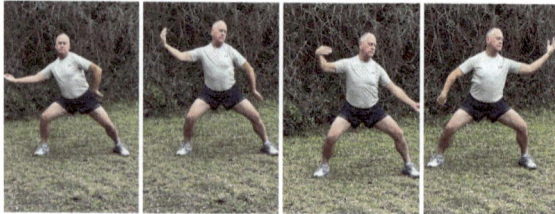

In a Horse Stance, with (L) hand on hip, (R) hand rises palm up, arm extended to side. Hand, palm down, thumb tucked when beside the body, moves to skim close to the body from shoulder to hip ending with palm to back. Turning palms back up repeat the circle 8 times. Reverse and repeat motion with (L) hand 8 times. With both hands, rising side palm up, and lowering side palm down, alternate hands and repeat 8 times.

Basically, scooping them up. Tuck the thumb as the hand comes underneath the shoulder. Now, instead of this being what I call a limb exercise, where all I am doing is using them, I am going to be able to turn from the waist. So, I am rooting for my left leg to come out through the right side.

Shake or Stir the Chi

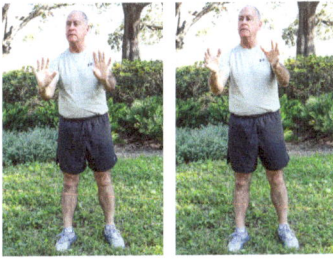

It is shaking the body. Shaking the fists. This is shaking or stirring the chi. I am slowing it down. I am going to turn from the waist so that there is a spiral going on in the legs, and you can be rolling the fists lightly here. Or you could be like pulling on something or punching against something. There is a forwards and backwards motion.

Begin in a Neutral Stance, feet apart, firmly rooted. Continue to do a cleansing movement. When the palms have come down in front of the chest reach out in front of the body as if catching the chi or energy in the air. ... Shake loosely. The waist and shoulders all move. (variation: roll forearms from embrace position, knuckles aligning in front of body.)

You want to twist the wrists and shake the chi in the palms. Turn the wrists. Loosening and relaxing let the arms go back down to the sides of the body. Begin the cleansing exercise 1 and Inhale the breath bringing the arms up allowing the fingertips to point directly up towards the sky like a funnel (Body forms a Y in shape), the hands come back towards each other creating a covering over the crown of the head. When the palms pass in front of the face, lower the tongue inside the mouth. As you exhale down. Then, the tongue returns to the roof of the mouth. Shifting weight into a neutral position stance.

Cleansing

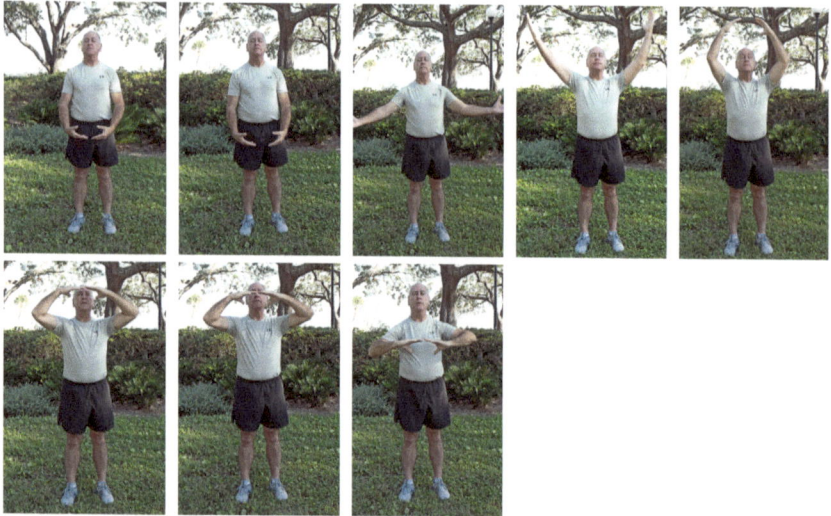

Repeat the opening movement, if necessary, read that section again.

Then, cleanse doing the cleansing breath and hands exercise. Bring the fingertips together palm up in front of the lower waist. Drawing up and bringing the fingertips to point to the sky then together over the head and then palms facing down over the crown of the head and gently press palms down in front of the body then press down to earth letting the hands/palms settle alongside the body.

Standing Meditation - 3 Hand Postures or Posts

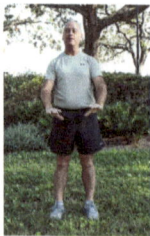
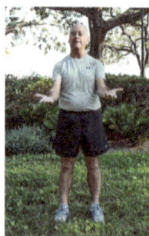
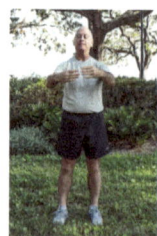

earth   sky-heaven   human-embrace

Begin in a Neutral Stance, knees slightly bent or relaxed, feet apart. Eyes are closed during this exercise if comfortable. Hands extended in front of hips, palms down (Earth). Hold posture for count of 8*; Transition by slowly turning palms up (Sky or Heaven). Hold for count of 8.

Transition by Lifting elbows, pointing fingers toward each other, but not touching; arms are rounded as though in an embrace (Human). Maintain roundness of circle, relax shoulders. Hold for count of 8.

NOTE: *if you want to do more advanced work or challenge these postures may be held for any amount of time up to 1 hour.*

Changing position into a Neutral stance do another cleansing

Closing

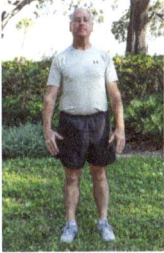

Shift weight right, slight bend of right knee.
Bring the left leg beside the right leg. Bow to close.

Wu Ji
emptying the mind meditation

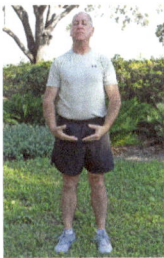

Begin with the heels together, knees slightly bent or relaxed "not locked," feet, toes slightly apart. Eyes are closed (if able or comfortable). Meditate by focusing mentally to lower dan tien. Focus on breathing from dan tien. Relax, yet maintain posture. Hold for count of 8.

advanced challenge: hold any posture for any amount of time, or up to 1 hour.

STANCES

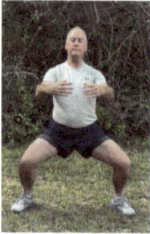

Horse Stance

Arms embracing form a large round circle in front of the body; fingertips point to one another without touching: To assume horse stance, start with heels together forming a 'V' or 45-degree angle, facing front.

Alternately move first heels, then toes out in a zigzag pattern five times, ending with heels. Feet are spread apart approximately twice one's shoulder width. Press heels slightly out, then lowers the body as though sitting on a saddle or edge of a chair. In the beginning, do not try to go any lower than it is comfortable.

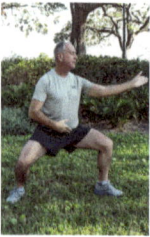 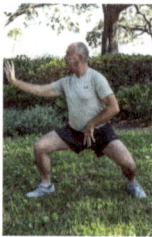

Bow Stance
right side forward & left side forward

Begin in Horse Stance, shift weight right, move left toes toward the center, pivot on the left heel. Place weight on (L) foot, turn waist, lift right toes, pivot on right heel, adjust (R) foot by rooting from (L) foot. (Advanced students, weight should be 60% on the right leg. Knee should be bent so "ideally" the right thigh is parallel to the ground.) (R) foot is toed in. The right knee does not go past the toes. The right palm extends away from the body, fingers point to the sky. Head is turned toward the (R) hand. Eyes look over the fingers lined up in a row. Extend the thumb and the index finger to create the "Tiger's Mouth."

(Optional, the eyes may look between the thumb and index finger, through the "Tiger's Mouth.") The (L) hand is drawn back as if on a bow. Extend fingers of (L) hand pointing to the earth, the thumb tucks at the dan tien or belt region. This completes Right Side Forward.

LEFT SIDE FORWARD: Using the same principles described, change to the other side. Reverse the placement of the feet and hands.

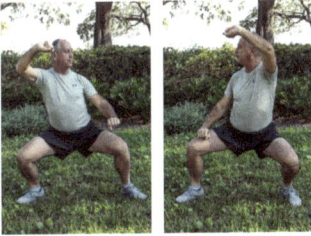

Back Stance

left side & right side

Feet shoulder width apart; feet flat to ground (can also be in lower posture or horse stance); knees bent; Weight on right side; Left toes point slightly left, right toes point forward; Right fist up, palm out, even with eyebrow, arms rounded, press away from body; left fist, palm down at hip level. Reverse by bringing left toes in, shift weight to left side and right toes point slightly right. Reverse first positions.

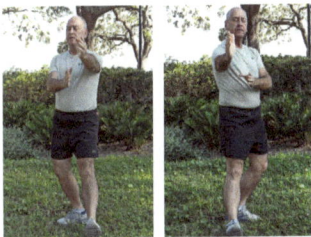

7-Star Stance or Play Guitar

left side & right side

Begin with the (L) foot forward with toes raised approximately 45* angle and the heel touching ground, (R) foot back, flat on ground, toes pointing to right, weight on the right side, slight natural bend in knees. Arms extended to front with natural bend at elbows, palms in. (L) hand forward, (R) hand slightly lower and back.

REVERSE - weight on left; (R) foot forward, toes up, heel touching ground, (L) foot back, flat, toes point left. (R) hand forward, (L) hand slightly lower and back.

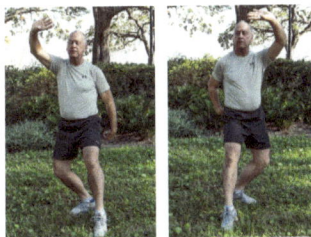

Cat Stance

left side & right side

Begin with the weight on the right side; (R) foot flat, pointing slightly right; knees slightly bent. (L) foot forward with only toes or ball of foot touching ground. Rounding the arms, (L) hand back, fingers. touching to form a point, (Crane's Beak) hooks behind back. (R) hand, palm out, pressing forward and away from the right eyebrow. Change Posture by placing (L) foot flat in Neutral Stance, shift weight to the left side. Extend (R) foot forward, toes touch ground, (R) hand, in Crane's Beak, hooks behind back. (L) hand, palm out, pressing forward and away from the left eyebrow.

Single Leg Stance

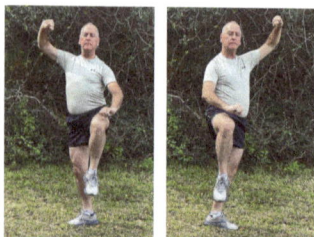

left side & right side
Begin with the weight on right side; (R) foot flat, pointing to right side; (L) foot forward with toes touching; Right fist pressing away from ear, extended above eyebrow; Left fist, palm down.

At hip level above left thigh, Slowly lift left knee and hold posture. Lower (L) foot and shift weight to left side. Reverse foot and hand positions; slowly lift right knee and hold. If it is not possible to lift your legs, hold stance using cat footwork instead. Changing position into a Neutral stance do another cleansing

Cleansing

Then, cleanse doing the cleansing breath and hands exercise. Bring the fingertips together palm up in front of the lower waist. Drawing up and bringing the fingertips to point to the sky then together over the head and then palms facing down over the crown of the head and gently press palms down in front of the body then press down to earth letting the hands/palms settle alongside the body. Complete the qigong routine by settling into a neutral position stance.

Wu Ji

Begin with the heels together and the feet are slightly apart forming a 'V' shape, face and eyes looking forward, arms relaxed at sides. Close eyes if comfortable, mentally focus on lower dan tien; breathing is full, relaxed, and natural originating from dan tien. Maintain a gentle relaxed focus and become aware.

Closing
Bow with Peace & Gratitude

concluding the practice session for now

ABOUT THE AUTHOR'S TEACHER

Master Frank J. Paolillo has studied with several of China's finest teachers.

He is a certified teacher (Sifu) of the Shantung Martial Arts of China and recipient of the "Educator of Kung Fu" award under his primary teacher:

• Grandmaster Pui Chan of Sha Cheng - Wah Lum Kung Fu.

In 1993, Sifu Paolillo assisted as coach of the U.S. Kung Fu Team at the World Championships held in Zhengzhou, China. He also served as Chief Judge of the Internal Martial Arts division at the 2000 World Championships held in Orlando, Florida. This competition is now known as the International Chinese Martial Arts Championship (ICMAC) established 1998.

Sifu Paolillo has studied with Internal Martial Arts Masters:

• Kay Chi Leung of Taiwan
• Li En Jiu of Jinan
• Zhang Xia Xin of Bejing
• Hing Ling Kwan of Zhengzhou (a student of Sha Guo Zheng).

Sifu Paolillo's instruction includes the cultivation of essence, chi (inner energy) & spirit through:

• Taoist meditation & qigong
• the silk-like reeling spiraling power movements of Chen tai chi chuan
• the coiling, twisting & circling movements of dragon baguazhang
• the speed & patience of northern praying mantis kung fu
• Chinese Shantung weapons training to further enhance awareness, agility, centering & manifestation of energy to power.

ABOUT THE AUTHOR

Paul began his formal training in martial arts in 1991 with Master F.J. Paolillo. In addition to silk reeling qigong, he has studied Chen style tai chi chuan, northern praying mantis, snake, dragon style baguazhang, various Shantung weapons such as: double-edged sword, broadsword, staff, spear, cane, kwan do, and other internal Taoist arts. Paul received permission from his "Sifu" to teach and has taught numerous tai chi and qigong classes since 1995.

Qualified by his Sifu F.J. Paolillo & by Grandmaster Pui Chan's authority he was a Tournament Official as a competition judge in kung fu, Chinese weapons, and tai chi at the Tournament 2000 International Kung Fu Championship in Orlando, Florida. This competition is now known as the International Chinese Martial Arts Championship (ICMAC) established 1998.

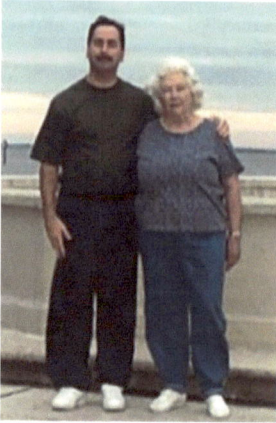

Paul Ellsworth & his student
Joyce C. Morris at Memorial Park
Jacksonville, FL year 2000.

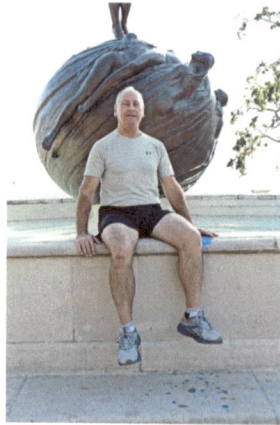

Paul Ellsworth at Memorial Park,
Jacksonville, FL January 2025.

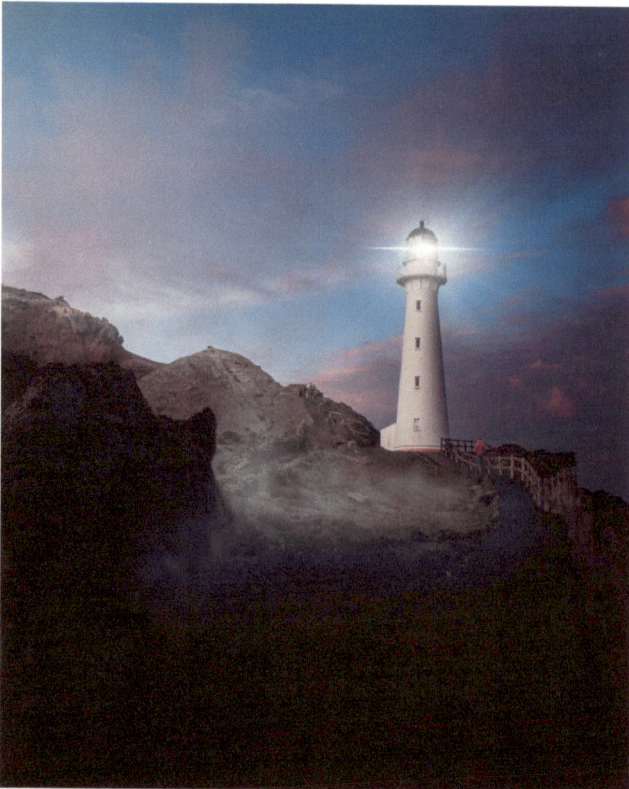

www.ingramcontent.com/pod-product-compliance
Lightning Source LLC
Chambersburg PA
CBHW041214270326
41930CB00001B/19